Praise for Robert W. Smith and
The Parkinson's Playbook

"Bob and his supporters define the extraordinary response to chronic illness. Applying the same collaborative creative approach that characterized his professional career, he is winning over his disease. *The Parkinson's Playbook* is an amazing journal of powerful and useful lessons learned. Go Bob!"

> —NAN ANDERSON, Principal, FAIA
> (Fellow of the American Institute of Architects)

"Bob's story of living with Parkinson's disease has been quite a journey; he is improving his life in coping with this unforeseen turn of events, and wants to help others take control of their lives. Way to go, Bob!"

> —JEAN SMITH, Spouse

"Bob's story is proof that our bodies and minds can heal themselves when they have what they need to do it. This book will transform many lives!"

> —AMANDA JOHNSON, True to Intention

"Robert Smith, you are an inspiration to so many! When you were my yoga student, I was continually amazed at your determination to stay strong, flexible and positive. Your story has the potential to help so many people with Parkinson's! I wish you love and blessings on your journey with *The Parkinson's Playbook*."
  —DEBORAH LONERGAN YATSKO

"I know Bob very well. He designed my Korean and WWII Memorials (in New Jersey). I saw him decline during those first years, and have had the joy of seeing him rebound. I had the opportunity to review the draft of *The Parkinson's Playbook* last year. If you have a connection to Parkinson's, you should take a look at this."
  —STEPHEN G. ABEL, Colonel, U. S. Army (Retired)

"*The Parkinson's Playbook* gives a new meaning to dedication and perseverance. It takes both, and more, to complete the game he so wonderfully describes as he accepts his fate as a "sweet victory" over Parkinson's. You are playing a great game, Bob, and belong in the Hall of Fame for your effort!"
  —DONALD GODI, FASLA (Fellow of the American
    Society of Landscape Architects)

"Bob's book is really impressive. His way of dealing with Parkinson's can really fit any chronic illness. I have been using some of his methods in dealing with my lung and heart disease. Keep on going, Bob."
  —JANE HULTIN

"Bob continually brought a high level of excellence to his work. As a leader, he pushed the boundaries of landscape architecture while promoting advancement of his whole team. I am proud of his efforts that he applied to addressing his Parkinson's that has helped him preserve his quality of life. This book is another example of Bob's interest in sharing his own achievements so that others can benefit from his hard work."

—ANN CHRISTENSEN, ASLA (American Society of Landscape Architects), Chief of Business Development, Managing Principal, DHM Design Corp.

"Bob, I was so moved at how many people were blown away by the changes they've seen in you. I'm happy to be a part of your team, but the biggest player here is YOU! Without your determination and dedication to facing this disease head-on every day, you would never have gotten this far. That takes a very strong and motivated person to keep at it day after day and not just take the easy route. I'm truly inspired by your progress, and I can only hope I get to work with people as determined as you throughout my career in medicine."

—ALANA FOELLER, Yoga Therapist, Ayurveda Practitioner, and Registered Nurse

"I have been Bob's massage therapist on and off since 2005. Upon his diagnosis, Bob appeared to begin having the onset of symptoms associated with Parkinson's, including tremors, cognitive difficulties, and physical difficulties walking. His proactive, holistic approach immediately began improving his overall health. Muscle tone has increased, weight has dropped to normal, and he has virtually no tremors. Along with all this, his strength and stamina have increased and, in turn, resulted in a more youthful and healthy appearance. He seems to be more balanced and jovial. Bob has a new lease on life, and I am thoroughly impressed and convinced this is the direction Parkinson's treatment should be going."

—ASHLEY RHINES, Massage Therapist

"Bob, I just read *The Parkinson's Playbook*, I got chills running up and down my arms as I read the introduction. I loved your book! What a gift this will be to so many people! You are truly a heroic role model...and your Playbook is inspirational providing hope, wisdom, and lessons for how to live life whether you have Parkinson's or not! I hope you go on to speak at seminars and conferences. You have so much to teach doctors, individuals with Parkinson's and their families, and all of us who don't have Parkinson's. Your journal is a must-read!"
    —MELANIE WELLER M.S., L.C.P.C. (Licensed Clinical
        Professional Counselor)

"As Robert's psychologist since 2010, I have witnessed the truly remarkable positive changes he made in his life to deal with the mental and emotional degradation brought on by Parkinson's. After several years of psychotherapy it seemed as if he was becoming younger with each passing day as the rest of us continued to age. Through dedication, self-reflection, and perseverance, he defined a path to a plateau of health from which he refused to stray. I am confident he will never lose sight of the fact that his current elevated level of comprehensive health and wellness is a result of his steadfast efforts and determination. It has been my good fortune to work with an individual possessing such inner strength and commitment."
    —J. MICHAEL FARAGHER, Psy.D. CACIII NCGC/BACC

THE PARKINSON'S PLAYBOOK

A Game Plan to Put Your Parkinson's on the Defense

ROBERT W. SMITH

Hatherleigh Press is committed to preserving and protecting the natural resources of the earth. Environmentally responsible and sustainable practices are embraced within the company's mission statement.

Visit us at www.hatherleighpress.com and register online for free offers, discounts, special events, and more.

THE PARKINSON'S PLAYBOOK

David Burnett, Bob's Broncos, Bowen Practitioner, International Institute of Bowen Studies. www.bowenstudies.org

Photo Credits
Photos courtesy of the Smith Family:
Robert Smith, Jean Smith, and Natalie Andl.
Yoga pose photos courtesy of Gwen Lawrence.
Bowen and SCENAR photos courtesy of David Burnett.

Library of Congress Cataloging-in-Publication Data is available upon request.
ISBN: 978-1-57826-708-8

COVER AND INTERIOR DESIGN BY CAROLYN KASPER

Printed in the United States

11

DISCLAIMER

This book is published with the understanding that the author and publisher are not engaged in rendering medical, health, or any kind of personal professional services in the book.

The information in this book describes the author's personal journey and is provided in good faith. It should not be considered to be complete or exhaustive regarding the topic it covers, and it is not intended to provide or be a substitute for professional medical or wellness advice or opinion or the basis for diagnosing, treating, curing, or preventing any disease or health condition. The reader should contact, consult, and discuss all medical or wellness issues with a qualified physician or physicians and/or health care professional or professionals familiar with the reader's particular circumstances. The information has not been evaluated by any governmental agency, physician, or health care provider or peer reviewed. Its use is entirely at the reader's risk.

This book contains the opinions and ideas of the author and associate contributors, none of who guarantee or warrant the validity of the information. It is intended to provide helpful and informative material on the subjects addressed in the book. The reader should understand that there can be differences of opinion and treatment concerning health care, and also note that changes and advances in medical practices as well as changes and developments in technology are factors that may impact information in this book. Furthermore, it is reasonable to believe and understand that all forms of treatment and treatment strategies and exercise programs carry some risk.

It should be noted that this book may contain outdated or incorrect information and that the publisher, author, and contributors may not update or correct and do not represent that they will update or correct. Any claims and or testimonials in this book are only anecdotal and should not be interpreted to be indicative of a reader's experience of health condition.

The author and the publisher disclaim all liability for damages caused by doing the lessons or applying the recommendations in this book.

The author, contributors, publisher, and everyone else involved in producing this book specifically disclaim and do not assume any responsibility or liability whatsoever, legal or otherwise, for any, loss, damage, injury, or risk, personal or otherwise, concerning the information, or errors, omissions, or inaccuracies in the information, and give no assurance regarding and shall not be responsible for the accuracy, completeness, usefulness of any information, apparatus, product, medicine, exercise, therapy, or process disclosed and/or discussed in this book or the consequences, directly or indirectly, of any action or actions taken on the basis of the information provided.

Further, the aforementioned persons make no warranty, representation, or undertaking whatsoever of any kind, either express or implied, regarding the information in this book and disclaim any warranty, representation, or undertaking whatsoever that may be expressed or implied by statute, custom or otherwise. In no event will the aforementioned persons be liable to the reader or any other person for any fees, cost, expense, or loss, whether direct, indirect, or incidental, or any punitive, exemplary, special, or consequential damages which may arise from use of the information in this book, whether arising out of a claimed breach of warranty or otherwise.

AUTHOR'S NOTE

T*he Parkinson's Playbook* is a story of my journey with a debilitating disease, from diagnosis, to denial, to a downward spiraling course of health and a life-changing path to a healthy and fulfilling lifestyle. The cornerstone of the "Game Plan" in this book is to leave no stone unturned in the pursuit of a higher quality of life. My program is a blending of traditional medicine (what we call "The Defense") and a holistic natural philosophy ("The Offense"), with unique treatment strategies that follows a never-before-traveled road for living with Parkinson's. It is a story of self-healing for both the body and mind that puts a chronic disease on the defense.

The Parkinson's Playbook is devoted to providing a ray of hope to those suffering with Parkinson's disease that, with commitment, can lead to a fuller and more vibrant life.

—ROBERT W. SMITH

ACKNOWLEDGMENTS

DAVID AND GAYLA BURNETT: Our dear friends, the Burnetts, developed a protocol to improve my quality of life and a path to deal with Parkinson's. Their first step was helping me to gain disability coverage, followed by the development of a program they created for me that we called "Bob's Broncos" (which ultimately became the launching point for *The Parkinson's Playbook*) that gave my family a process for self-healing. They put forth a challenge at every step of the journey, with enough latitude so that I could still enjoy my life.

MY FAMILY, JEAN SMITH AND NATALIE ANDL: I cannot say enough how grateful I am for Jean and Natalie's help in dealing with Parkinson's every day. They have seen me at my highs and lows, but never wavered in their support. I am not sure I could have made the changes from being in the throes of Parkinson's to improving my quality of life without their help.

ALANA FOELLER: Alana was at the core of my ability to slow down Parkinson's with yoga therapy and her expertise in developing a fitness program. As you follow my journey, you will see Alana's skill in formulating a comprehensive plan that allowed me to remain active (biking, skiing, and walking), which is imperative for anyone with Parkinson's. Alana became a part of the Smith family with her dedication and loyalty.

J. MICHAEL FARAGHER: Mike played an important role as my psychologist, providing me with the tools for fighting depression, anxiety, and stress. His approach was not to simply give me advice, but to help me find my own answers and understand how to cope with the many facets of Parkinson's. We would talk about an issue and how to resolve it, which enabled me to take an active role and ownership to change my life for the better.

AMANDA JOHNSON: Amanda brought life to *The Parkinson's Playbook,* transforming a rough manuscript into an engaging story that needs to be shared and is relevant to those dealing with Parkinson's and other chronic diseases. Amanda was integral in shaping the story of my journey with Parkinson's. She was much more than an editor and coach, but a team member who could weave together the many treatment strategies for Parkinson's into a comprehensive guidebook.

CONTENTS

FOREWORD

Shortly before the completion of this book, I had lunch with Bob Smith and our colleague, Jeff Shoemaker. Bob brought some drawings, photos, and memorabilia recounting the revitalization of the South Platte River in Denver. Over several decades, the three of us have worked, in our respective professions, to engage in transforming what was once a lost and blighted landscape into a major new green amenity. As a multi-faceted and visionary landscape architect, Bob played a lead role in inspiring the transformation that many thought was impossible.

As the three of us mused about how the South Platte was now flourishing and invigorating the surrounding communities, I couldn't help but make the comparison to how Bob has faced the challenge of Parkinson's disease. When diagnosed in 2006, he faced a daunting medical and personal trial—a test that would cause many to retreat. Instead, he decided to take this trial head-on; to fight back, to will a different course for his life in much the same way that he and others willed a different outcome for our compromised river.

As Bob was perfecting his draft of this book, he asked me—as a friend and an author, having been a reviewer for Island Press and others—to review and critique his writing. When first asked, I had doubts that I would be of any substantive value because I do not have Parkinson's disease. Those doubts, however, vanished once I started reading Bob's amazing reflections, quickly realizing that this is a "playbook" that has value to anyone facing any and every kind of life challenge. In reality, Bob's book is a guide—both practical and inspiring—about adapting and making an enduring comeback. It chronicles the challenge of living with a formidable adversity and, more importantly, living well! Bob's reflections are about how to navigate a host of difficulties—personal, medical, and emotional—that virtually all of us are facing, or will face.

It is to be read and kept as a way-finding tool!

As we finished lunch, Jeff shared a story about a closet in his office. He said it was full of a bunch of items that came over from a recent move, and he laughed about how everyone in the office avoided opening the door, knowing it would mean facing the challenge of putting order into the disarray. He said, "There are times when we all can use some guidance to enter that closet, take on chaos, and bring back the calm that comes in restructuring for the better."

I smiled as I looked at the now nearly-symptom-free Bob and realized that this is what he's done for the readers who pick up this book.

If you or someone you know suffers with Parkinson's, *The Parkinson's Playbook* will give you what you need to take on the chaos of this disease, bring some peace into the process, and restructure your life and health for the better.

—ROBERT SEARNS, AICP (American Institute of Certified Planners), author of *Greenways:, A Guide to Planning, Design, and Development*

PREFACE

As a practitioner of Internal Medicine, I have overseen Robert Smith's health care since 1981, when he was an active, healthy, vibrant, productive, and incredibly talented landscape architect. He had the occasional mild illnesses many of us experience from time to time. Late in 2005, he began noticing shaking in his right upper extremity which seemed to be steadily progressing. A referral to a neurologist resulted in a diagnosis of Parkinson's disease. This devastating diagnosis would challenge him mentally, physically, and socially. It would forever change Robert's life, impacting all aspects of his living and causing him to abandon his very successful career in 2011.

Neither his physicians nor Robert knew how he would confront this illness, characterized by profound symptoms of fatigue, tremor, impaired gait, depression, and changes in physical appearance. He attacked the disease head-on, to not only regain a healthy perspective on life both mentally and physically, but also to make it his mission to help others understand the many debilitating aspects of this disease with the publication of *The Parkinson's Playbook*.

Robert's journey was anything but easy and was littered with many setbacks and episodic disease progression. In early 2011, Robert began an upward climb in health and fitness, which sparked a goal to produce a playbook for people living with Parkinson's. His check-ups the past few years have been rather remarkable, with steady improvement to what would be considered a normal report card. He remains alert, intellectually engaged, and physically very active. If you were not aware of his history, you would not know that he has Parkinson's disease. At his most recent exam, it was evident that his exercise program and mental attitude are having a profound impact in his success dealing with this difficult disease.

It has been a joy to witness firsthand Robert's hard work, commitment, and tenacity to keep pace with Parkinson's, let alone author and publish a book of this significance. I am honored to be part of Robert's health care team.

—STANLEY J. KERSTEIN, MD, FACP, Denver Internal Medicine

THE GAME OF YOUR LIFE

"Some people think football is a matter of life and death. I assure you, it's much more serious than that." —BILL SHANKLY

Every player sits upright when the coach walks in. They are only a few minutes away from beginning the biggest, most important game of the season—and of some of the players' entire lives. Silence, tension, and a ton of adrenaline courses through the room.

"This is it, men. In a few minutes, you are going to stand face-to-face with your most formidable opponent yet. But you've been working hard for this moment all season. All the drills, all the new plays, all of the long hours—it was all to get you here and prepare you for this game. This is the game of your life. Play hard. Play smart. Play proud."

The team echoes his words, "Play hard. Play smart. Play proud," back to him and to each other, anchoring their common intention and energy to defeat the team that awaited them on the field.

THE DIAGNOSIS

This is a nightmare! Get me out of here!

Strapped down by my legs, chest, arms, and head on a white slab of plastic, I started to panic in the cold, isolated tube. The shock of the experience of the last few hours and days set off a rapid-fire, movie-like experience, making it very hard for me to not lose my mind in that god-awful tube.

The doctor and MRI staff acted like this wasn't going to be a big deal. How could he say that he thinks I have Parkinson's when he just looked at my hand?

"Mr. Smith, stop moving. We're almost there." One of the nurses tried to calm me down.

I can't stop shaking! How can they flippantly diagnose me with Parkinson's because of a tremor and then expect me to control it while I'm in the tube?!

"Get me out of here!" I screamed at the top of my lungs, unable to hide the fear and desperation coursing through me. I felt like I was going to explode. It wasn't just the cold, claustrophobic tube . . .

This is a death sentence, isn't it? I mean, people with Parkinson's just get worse and worse, and then die. Will I never have a normal life again?

The reality, or maybe I should say the *gravity*, of my situation finally hit me.

When my wife noticed the shaking in my right arm and hand for the first time a few weeks before, we were watching television, and she simply said, "Maybe you should see your doctor about that." That was it. The thought of Parkinson's never even entered our minds.

And then the doctor. In twenty minutes, he told me to find a neurologist and tell them everything I'd just shared with him. No mention of Parkinson's. Just an urgency to find a neurologist (at random, it seemed) and have them check me out.

But then the neurologist immediately diagnosed it as Parkinson's,

"The tremors of the left arm, shuffling gait, and lack of facial expression—telltale signs of Parkinson's."

As the first step, the neurologist felt I should have an MRI to confirm it.

I did not have a clue what an MRI is and what it would be like. The MRI staff casually prepared me for the exam, and I never thought I would have a problem with it. Somehow, I thought it would be similar to getting an x-ray at the dentist's office.

And now I'm in hell. Get me out!

I tried to force myself free, but it was useless.

Why are they continuing when I am going nuts?

When they finally let me out and unstrapped me, I left the building and got to my car as quickly as I could.

What am I supposed to do now? Go home? Go back to work like nothing happened?

(Comment: If you ever have an MRI, ask the doctor for a sedative prior to starting the procedure.)

At the follow-up appointment, the neurologist showed me the negatives, which in itself was a frightening experience. Then he said something that shocked me, "I didn't think the MRI would show anything anyway. Parkinson's usually doesn't show up on these tests." And then he handed me the negatives and said, "You should keep these."

In hindsight, I can see how inappropriate it was to treat a person like that when they have just recently been diagnosed with Parkinson's disease, but he also took for granted that I knew everything there was to know about it.

That was the first sign that I was alone on this Parkinson's path.

(Comment: As I am typing this, my right leg has tremors from just the emotion of telling my diagnosis story. I had to stop and let it calm down. The fear still sits with me today.)

BIG LOSSES TO BIG WINS

I was diagnosed with Parkinson's in January of 2006 and became one of the more than 1.5 million Americans afflicted with the disease. In fact, there are 60,000 new cases diagnosed annually.

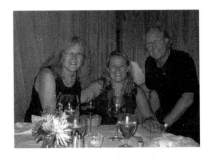

The Smith Family, 2006

Working 60 to 80 hours per week while being treated for the disease was limiting my ability to make positive changes in my life. I was taking the treatment lightly, not wanting to believe that I had a debilitative disease without a known cure. Each year, the symptoms were progressing faster, with right arm tremors, poor balance, shuffling gait, nausea from the medications, and rigidity of my trunk and arms. As time progressed, depression, stress, and anxiety were compounding the already debilitating course of Parkinson's.

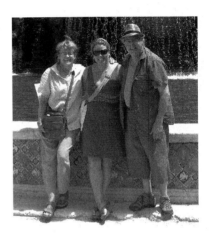

The Smith Family, 2010

From 2006 to 2010, I followed the traditional path of Parkinson's medications as the main direction for stabilizing my condition. It was a struggle to deal with the side effects of the medications. The combination of Parkinson's pills coupled with depression, anxiety, and stress would bring on nausea and light-headedness for several hours, until the drugs went through my system. I was losing one-third of my day adjusting to the side effects of all the medications.

After four years of struggling on my own with Parkinson's and its associated complications, I was on a spiraling decline in health and emotional wellness. By the fall of 2010, I was at a turning point. There were only two paths to take: I could either let Parkinson's take over my life, or I could admit that even my best "defense" using traditional medicine wouldn't be enough to stop the disease, and instead choose to go on the "offense," finding *new* ways to push Parkinson's back and down.

I was fortunate to have friends with a background in health care and self-healing. The Burnetts, David and Gayla (who practice Bowen Therapy, focused on drug-free pain relief) stepped in to share their knowledge based on many years of experience in the healthcare field.

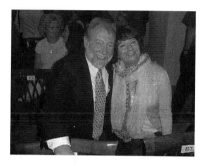

David and Gayla Burnett

In my opinion, the Burnetts created the most comprehensive wellness health plan ever compiled for dealing with Parkinson's disease.

They spent months developing an all-inclusive program to give me the tools to fight this debilitating disease. When you search the web, there is a lot of information on the technical evaluation of Parkinson's, but there is not a definitive tried-and-true path you can take. You need someone to connect the dots. It would have been impossible for me to come up with an approach with my ever-decreasing mental capacity.

Their first step was to help me apply for three-year disability coverage through my place of work. The interesting part is that after you apply and receive approval, you go through it again with their evaluation company for a total of four applications plus Social Security Disability. With the Burnetts' help, I was able to gain approval in six weeks, a feat unheard of in the insurance world. I stopped work in February of 2011, and have used the past several years of disability coverage to make changes in my life.

My priority shifted to healing myself and not letting Parkinson's take over my life, but I'm not one to make changes easily with my stuck-in-the-mud attitude.

However, the Burnetts knew I was a Broncos fan and knew it would take a health plan that I could relate to and follow, so they created a fun health plan which they called "Bob's Broncos," which gave me a starting point with daily steps and direction. This plan later served as the foundation for *The Parkinson's Playbook*.

WHAT DO I MEAN BY A FAN?

A FAN is a person who only reads the Sports section!

A FAN calls in sick to watch the team practice in August when it's 95 degrees in the shade. Four thousand fans were at the practice session recently. These are serious fans.

A FAN always has a tailgate party with brats, burgers, green chili, and anything with beans.

A FAN gives the business to anyone who sells their tickets to the opposing team, especially rivals.

A FAN never misses a game, even when it's raining or snowing.

A FAN picks up their tickets the first day they are available at the stadium. (A FAN does not trust the Postal Service!)

A FAN goes to the exhibition games, even though they don't mean a damn thing.

A FAN has a shrine.

A FAN has a scale model of the old and new stadium, with a toothpick ready to show where your seats are.

A FAN has empty boxes of Eddie Mac's macaroni & cheese and Wheaties with John Elway's picture in their shrine.

A FAN wears their Eddie Mac jersey when they go skiing and chants, "Eddie! Eddie! Eddie!"

A FAN owns figurines of players from their champion years.

A FAN can name all of the players in the team's Ring of Fame.

A FAN high-fives other fans across the aisle.

A FAN, after twenty years, knows the names of the people sitting around them because they are all *fans*.

PLAY BY PLAY

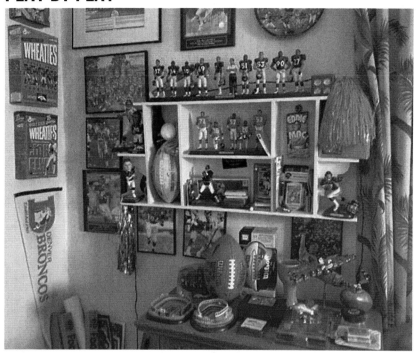

The Shrine

After stepping back from my career, it took a year to focus my energies and achieve my short-term goal of being fit. I suddenly had the energy necessary to make a difference in slowing down Parkinson's progression. It didn't take long to get a good handle on the physical fitness part. The motto, "Leave no stone unturned in the pursuit of a better quality of life," became the cornerstone of my new approach to Parkinson's and to life.

There are many physical and psychological obstacles to overcome on a daily basis. It has not been easy to stay on track. Parkinson's is a nasty disease, and it is relentless in pulling you down. From a physical standpoint, I have kept pace with the disease's effort to constantly erode my condition. The treatment strategies that I follow (which are laid out in this book) are very effective in improving my quality of life, but I can never slow down. When I speak about the commitment it takes to follow a fitness program, it is hard work to stay ahead in the game. The amount of effort I have devoted to exercise over the past four years equates to about 2,000 hours, or 500 hours a year, which is significant. The added benefit of the exercise regime is a body fat percentage of 14.9, indicating a lean body. It is so easy to back-track when you reach a high level of fitness, because you naturally feel you deserve a day off. But when you have Parkinson's, you cannot let that happen. Everyday fitness needs to be a part of your mindset.

THE FIRST PLAYBOOK

The Burnetts created a game plan uniquely tailored for me, and following the principles and strategies in that playbook has changed my life—it saved me in the most real sense possible. My Parkinson's is pretty stable at this point. I am fit and able to enjoy life within the confines of this illness. In fact, today, many people say, "I never would have known that you have Parkinson's."

The strategy was to build an offense that was just as powerful as the other team's defense, as well as an outstanding defense to keep our offense on the field longer. The goal, of course, is to score and maintain a lead over the other team on the scoreboard, and see measurable improvements by the end of every quarter. Finally, our team needed game-breaking players on both sides of the ball. In other words, we needed as many All Stars on our team as possible. Game-breaking players are a must when the score is close and we have to make the play or lose the ball.

WRITING THE BOOK

It took two years to put together *The Parkinson's Playbook*, and I often wondered if this was going to help people with Parkinson's disease, but I just kept thinking about how I felt in 2010 and how desperate I was for help. I had to help others.

Once we started to see really incredible results with my symptoms, we began talking about the possibility of sharing this game plan with others dealing with Parkinson's—those who fear that having Parkinson's disease is a death sentence and believe there is no way to stop the debilitative progression that shortens one's lifespan. I truly believe this book will not only inspire hope, but is designed to give you the specific principles, plays, strategies, and steps that will greatly improve your life.

We have a friend of more than thirty years who lives in Wisconsin and was just recently diagnosed with Parkinson's. He knew what I was up against and how I have been successful in slowing down the disease, and asked me to send him the list of supplements I take, which I did. A week later, I felt he needed more than a list of supplements, so I sent him the most recent draft of this book. Soon after, he called to say he downloaded it, printed it, and put it in a binder. He has read it three times (even though it was an early draft) and now has a powerful offense in place. He is losing weight, shuffles less, rides his bike, and stands taller.

I was truly amazed and am inspired that I am able to share this amazing game plan with you and others dealing with this horrible disease.

With the Burnett's permission, I have included most of the original playbook they designed for me (indicated by the pages with a gray border), in addition to sharing my own story and lessons learned. It's important to me that you know that what you are about to read is a careful blend of the Burnett's amazing expertise, my story, and what we have learned on this journey.

A PLAYBOOK FOR PARKINSON'S

It's probably apparent to you by now that I love football, and having a "playbook" that was deliberately connected to one of my passions made it easy for me to understand and more exciting to stick to.

I realize that others may not love football as much as I do, so while I use a lot of football jargon, I've done my best to stick to the basics of any sport in the hopes that anyone can connect the ideas to their favorite pastime and make faster strides, as I did.

I've also included some note-taking space, so that you can actually personalize your own playbook as you read. For example, after I share about the coaches and players I have on my defense, there will be some space for you to write down the names of doctors and coaches you already have or want to get on your team. I also recommend that you get a journal or begin one on your computer.

By the end of this book, you'll have your own personalized plan to improve your health and get into the end zone as often as you can to score the most points and win.

It will *really* help you to write down your specific goals, review them regularly, capture your successes on paper or in pictures, and really be able to see how far you've come.

So, grab a journal, and let's get started!

FIRST QUARTER
START WITH DEFENSE

"It's not whether you get knocked down, it's whether you get back up." —VINCE LOMBARDI

They all huddle around the coach, who is outlining the first few plays of the game.

"The key for this first quarter is defense," he says. "We have to see how this team is going to play this game. I've seen hours of video from their last few games and, if they play the same way here, we better have our defense ready. They come out swinging."

He looks up from his tablet and into the eyes of every player. "Just defense. Hold your ground. Don't give them an inch, and push them back where you can. You got it?"

All the eyes looking back at him gleam with hope that this will be their best game ever.

Seeing all heads nodding in understanding, the coach puts his hand in and waits for all of them to follow his lead before saying, "Let's go out and beat the crap out of these guys."

THE FIRST VISIT

"Okay, here's a prescription for your medications. Let's set an appointment for next month and see how those help reduce the tremors and slow down the disease."

"Okay. Will do." I answered quickly, feeling relieved that was all that I had to remember to do.

Life was getting harder to manage every day.

The less stress, the better, I thought to myself as I watched the doctor scribble notes in his chart.

In the course of a normal day, tremors in my right arm were not significant and were barely noticeable. However, when I was placed in a stressful situation, the tremors accelerated at an unbelievable rate. As if someone had flipped a switch, they would hit me by surprise and quickly become extremely difficult to conceal. Trust me, I tried to calm myself down and hide the shaking; but it was impossible, especially with the significant projects I was dealing with at work.

As a landscape architect, presentations were a major part of my job. I was the guy sent in to persuade and work with the often-difficult decision-makers (the "head honchos") on projects like new visitor facilities at Mount Rushmore National Memorial and Columbine Memorial, the Restoration of Giant Forest in Sequoia National Park, and a World War II Memorial for the state of New Jersey. It was the new visitor facility at Mather Point Grand Canyon National Park that was kicking my butt.

That last meeting about the project was awful.

I nodded back at the doctor and watched him leave the room to find sample medications before letting out the breath I had been holding for . . . I don't know how long?

I think I'm going to have to ask the guys on my team to help me get through the presentations. I don't want to tell them, but I just don't want to deal with client questions about why my hand shakes and why I'm using a podium like a fort or barrier to block the view of my shaking body.

Shaking my head at the thought, I walked out of the room and into a life that was feeling worse and worse every day, with very little hope for improvement.

He said these might be able to take care of the symptoms. That doesn't sound very promising.

THE OPPOSING TEAM: PARKINSON'S

Parkinson's disease (PD) is a chronic nervous system disorder that affects the brain, with subtle symptoms that worsen over time. It is a degenerative neurological disorder caused by an ever-decreasing supply of the brain chemical dopamine. While recent efforts have resulted in dramatic improvements in the treatment of its symptoms, there is still no known cure.

PD attacks the *substantia nigra*, the part of the brain that normally produces dopamine. Dopamine sends information to the parts of the brain that control muscles, movement, and coordination. When there is insufficient dopamine, the brain loses its ability to coordinate motor skills. This results in tremors (hands, arms, legs, and trunk), muscle rigidity, slowness of movement, difficulties with walking and balance, and reduced facial expressions. The brain may remain keen, knowing what it wants to do, but the message gets lost or confused.

Most Parkinson's patients begin to slowly develop tremors, difficulty balancing, stiff limbs, or slower movements in their fifties; the overwhelming majority of the 1.5 million Americans with the disease are in their sixties and beyond. The number of Americans afflicted is expected to triple over the next decades as the U.S. population ages.

Early symptoms of Parkinson's are diagnosed in stages, and can be so subtle and varied that the disease may go unnoticed for years. Since it takes time to develop the obvious motor symptoms, such as hand tremors, early detection is essential to confirm the correct diagnosis and initiate treatment. When there is a family history of the disease, it is important to inform one's health professionals so they can look for any possible early indicators.

DISORIENTING PLAYS AND SYMPTOMS

I was diagnosed with Parkinson's disease in 2006. In reality, the early symptoms were present for several years prior, but were not that noticeable. The common belief is that there are several early signs to help recognize Parkinson's. The early signs are generally associated with non-motor symptoms. There are many other symptoms, which may be part of your particular condition. In hindsight, the non-motor symptoms I noticed over time included:

- Speaking in a soft voice
- Speech issues (slurring, hesitation, or speaking monotonously)
- Difficulty finding words
- Continual constipation
- Waking up several times during the night
- Tightness of the ligaments in the balls of my feet
- Painful foot cramps
- Behavioral changes in personality
- Increased urination urgency/frequency
- Drooling
- Erectile dysfunction

DISABLING PLAYS AND SYMPTOMS

As dopamine in the brain decreases, Parkinson's symptoms progressively increase, affecting movement and muscle control and making the symptoms more noticeable. The first visible symptom for me was tremors of the right arm.

My motor symptoms were associated on the right side of my body, specifically my right arm. Motor symptoms I have experienced include the following:

- Tremors: trembling in the hands, arms, or legs
- Muscle rigidity: stiffness of the limbs and body
- Poor balance
- Slow movements
- Difficulty smiling and blinking
- "Masked" face, or a lack of expression
- Shuffling gait
- Trouble rising from seated position
- Difficulty swallowing
- Stooped posture and/or impaired balance
- Decreased arm swinging when walking
- Small handwriting
- Freezing, or walking in quick small steps

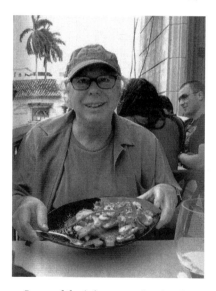

Loss of facial expression/smile

DAILY STRUGGLES

People with Parkinson's often combat significant cognitive impairments, which interfere with thinking, memory, and the ability to pay attention, solve problems, or make quick decisions. Some changes may be less obvious because they occur gradually. Some of the cognitive issues I experienced are listed below.

- General Functions: Trouble forming concepts, making plans, or reaching goals.
- Slowed Thinking: Typical daily tasks are challenging; problems are more difficult to solve. Following directions, as in recipes, is more difficult. (To help combat this, I have taken up cooking as a part of my household duties. So far, my specialties are asparagus soup, eggplant Parmesan, chili rellenos, and poblano peppers stuffed with mashed potatoes and cheese. Following recipes and making meals is rewarding as long as you are not counting calories.)
- Impaired Memory: Difficulty remembering information.
- Difficulty Paying Attention: Difficulty following complex scenarios, such as fully understanding a multi-person conversation.
- Symptoms of dementia, confusion, depression, and anxiety.

PARKINSON'S PLAY PROGRESSION

Although Parkinson's disease is categorized in five stages, its progression is individualized. This is especially true as advancements in treatment effectively slow its course. It is not uncommon to skip stages, or to have a variety of non-motor, motor, cognitive, and psychological symptoms at the same time. The pace at which the disease worsens also varies greatly. Diminishing cognitive impairments also track with each stage of Parkinson's. Treatments that I have been utilizing, including medications, supplements, exercise, and lifestyle changes, have effectively slowed the disease's progression. I am probably in Stage 2 as the Playbook is published.

- Stage 1: motor symptoms are confined to one side of the body
- Stage 2: motor symptoms appear on both sides of the body, but balance remains intact
- Stage 3: balance becomes more challenging
- Stage 4: motor functions are severely disabled but walking independently is still possible
- Stage 5: wheelchair-bound or bedridden

THE PARKINSON'S DRAFT: HOW DID I GET IT?

Often, Parkinson's folks are asked the question: "How did you contract Parkinson's?" It is not easy to come up with an answer. There is no specific known cause, which can leave a person searching for an answer. It's not like you can say, "I have a broken arm," and then the body heals itself and you are back to being your old self. Parkinson's is a chronic disease that has a life of its own. It is a progressive deterioration of your health. The disease surfaces slowly. In my case, it was not until my early sixties (generally fifty to sixty is considered a young age) when many of my symptoms appeared. The disease first surfaced with tremors on my right side. There are many variations of Parkinson's, but the bottom line is the body produces less dopamine, which has an impact on your nervous system and movement.

When I was diagnosed with Parkinson's disease, I tried to identify the root cause of the disease. The symptoms were easily found on the Internet, but they only seemed like a menu associated with Parkinson's. I realized, going down the list, that I was experiencing many of them. It was like a checklist of *I have this one* or *I don't have this one.* My issues centered on tremors, rigidity, balance, depression, anxiety, and stress.

Reviewing my symptoms in this way, with my wife's input, solidified the opinion that my Parkinson's was likely the result of detrimental environmental influences ranging from fertilizers, pesticides, and lawn weed killers to fumes from magic markers. There is no documented proof—it is just our opinion. The timeline below not only discusses the possible origin of my contracting Parkinson's but other significant points that influenced my journey with it.

One other thought as you read *The Parkinson's Playbook*: people with Parkinson's often repeat things so it sticks in their brain. As you come across this in the text, remember that it is a natural condition of the disease.

High School Years: 1962 to 1965

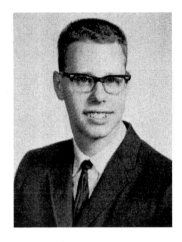

When I was 16 and a sophomore in high school, my main desire was to have a car (set of wheels), but my parents did not have the resources to buy a car. My first job, after school and on weekends, was at the local garden center and nursery close to school, so I was able to walk to work. Starting out at $0.50 an hour, I was able to buy my first car after saving up $200 for a 1956 Ford black convertible with a white top. It was hot stuff, but needed work!

The garden center specialized in plant material (annuals, perennials, shrubs, and trees), lawn fertilizer, landscape design and construction, pesticides, and a produce stand. We often would have our lunch on a stack of fertilizer. There were also times when we sold nasty stuff, like DDT. In the fertilizer area, there was a smell that permeated the room, which we got used to over time. Thinking back to that period of time, it was common to not realize the health dangers in the workplace. The detrimental environmental issues would not be allowed in this day and age. Yet there were good things about working at the garden center. It was where the manager, a landscape designer for the design/building part of the landscape business, introduced me to a career in landscape architecture.

College Years: 1965 to 1970

There were not any specific links to Parkinson's during my college years, but there could be a link to the tools a landscape architect used to render drawings. In school, we explored several graphic techniques, including markers, colored pencils, watercolors, caulk, and several others as part of our training. This was my first exposure to Xylene-based markers, which are now known to cause impairment to the central nervous system, with symptoms such as headache, dizziness, nausea, and vomiting. We also used spray adhesives, which have similar health issues and may cause eye, skin, nose, and throat irritation.

Landscape Architecture Practice: 1970's & 1980's

During this period, my career centered on designing park and recreation projects and involved preparing large plans for public presentations. Xylene markers were used extensively to produce illustrations that the general public could understand. The marker use did not seem to be an issue at that time, since they were used throughout the profession.

I was also required to lead large public presentations, which created a high level of anxiety. I would be shaking thinking about being in the spotlight. There were times when the only relief from anxiety was to throw up. I am not sure if it pointed to Parkinson's, or if it was just a part of working in the public eye.

DEFENSE: TRADITIONAL MEDICAL TEAM AND OPTIONS

David and Gayla Burnett

Your Defensive Goal

The key to the defensive game plan is to minimize the amount of time spent on defense. Your defense is on the field in response to the opposition's offense being on the field, playing with *your* ball! That's not good. The potential is that every time the opposition has the ball, you are at their mercy. You are playing by their rules, playing their tune. Do you want to suffer? Do you want to be dealing with symptoms? Do you want your quality of life to suffer? Are you going to be intimidated by their offense? Do you want it to be worse than it has to be? It doesn't have to be! The best and most effective form of defense is aggressive, in your face, where every down is their last play! It's critical to get the defense working for you, to use every tool (down) at your disposal to minimize the risk of them scoring and to get their offense off the field *now*!

Defensive Line: Your Medical Team

The foundation or baseline of every great defense is the effectiveness of the defensive line and its ability to put pressure on the offense, to create turnovers with sacks, fumbles, quarterback hurries, hand-offs, dropped passes, and even blocked punts and field goals.

The consequences of not having the optimal defensive line are far-ranging and impact your overall ability to fight this unrelenting foe. The results to date have been painful and potentially life threatening. This is about *you*, not them. Don't be shy about trying different doctors to find one that is right for you—keep looking until you find the right fit.

The Defensive Medical Team

Head Defensive Coach
(General Practitioner/Internal Medicine)

The role of your general practitioner is to monitor your overall health and track your medical condition with regular checkups (it also helps if they have current magazines in the lobby to read while waiting for your appointment). Even before being diagnosed with Parkinson's, this is the coach who tracks your blood pressure, cholesterol, prostate, and colon. Routine blood tests are taken as part of your annual exam. Essentially, he is your watchdog when it comes to your overall health and well-being

Assistant Defensive Coach (Neurologist)

The role of your neurologist is to formulate the best combination of medications to lessen symptoms (tremors) and to slow the progression of the disease. They also deal with the side effects brought on by the Parkinson's medication, including depression, anxiety, compulsive behavior traits, and stress. The neurologist is the key coach from the traditional medical field.

Mental Health Coach (Psychologist)

The mental and emotional experience of having Parkinson's is the hardest to wrap your hands around. The psychologist's role is to help you sort out the layers of depression that clog up your mental and behavioral health, and provide the therapy to deal with anxiety and stress. They are the Most Valuable Player (MVP) on your Parkinson's team.

Special Teams Coach (Counselor)

The counselor provides advice and guidance in the search for professionals that are experienced in working with Parkinson's patients. They are the best person to coordinate and manage the defense's game plan. You don't have to like this doctor/counselor—it's not about their bedside manner or if they run to take time off of the clock. It's about who is best qualified and able to run a modern, up-to-the-minute, effective, and efficient defense. They are "ruthless" at minimizing the ability of the opposing offense to gain ground. They are plugged into the right organizations to know the latest medications, the drugs being tested, and the latest "hot" technique.

NEUROLOGIST SESSION

While I was waiting for my appointment with the neurologist, I would often scan the room for others, trying to pick out those with Parkinson's and their stage of debilitation. One day, there was a guy on the other side of the room shaking like a leaf, hunched over in a wheelchair.

Oh my goodness. I could be that guy soon! My stomach sank at the idea.

Almost as soon as the doctor walked into the room, I asked him, "Am I going to look like the guy in the waiting room?"

He smiled and said, "He has something entirely different!"

Phew. There is hope for me.

Office Visit Experience

Below are the top 10 questions and happenings at each appointment with the neurologist:

#1: It's time for my appointment, they call out my name and scan the room. *This would be a good time to be a ghost so I could avoid talking about my condition.*

#2: "Let me see you walk down the hall." *It's like being a model on the runway. I may fall if I try the catwalk, though!*

#3: The doc reviews the form. *Looks like he's having trouble making heads or tails of my handwriting!*

#4: "Hold out your hands, squeeze my hand, relax your hands—you have signs of arthritis!" *Oh good, just want I want to hear!*

#5: "Are you depressed?" *What do you think? I have Parkinson's and now you're telling me I have arthritis?*

#6: "Do you have any compulsive habits?" *Ummm . . . why do you ask?*

#7: "Do you have Erectile Dysfunction? Do you want Viagra?" *I doubt my wife does. Up to four hours is a long time for anyone!*

#8: "You misspelled Parkinson's." *Have you seen me write?*

#9: "Is this written in an ancient language?" *Ummm . . . has someone told you I have Parkinson's? It means my hand shakes A LOT.*

#10: "Let's meet in three months to see how you are dealing with your medications!" *I wish I was cured!*

WAITING FOR YOUR APPOINTMENT

The biggest pain in the butt is filling out the update form at each visit. I am usually sitting in a chair with only my leg and a clipboard for a writing surface. The top part of the form asks for information about who you are and who your doctors are, and half the time I misspell one of the names of a doctor. The second section is to list *all* of your medications.

How in the world can you remember all your drugs and their dosage? Impossible!!!

It's like learning a new language. Now I bring a printed list and ask the front desk to staple it to the form. One issue resolved!

The third section asks about your issues, and man, they can see one of my biggest issues just by trying to read my writing. My longhand stinks, I misspell a lot of words, there are cross-outs everywhere, and often I turn the chart sideways and write in the margin. I've learned over time that just listing your medical complaints is depressing. After writing about my problems, I draw a line and list happy thoughts!

The following chart will give you a sense of how I deal with forms while waiting to see the doctor. It gives you an idea why the doctor needs a magnifying glass to read your small lettering and understand what you are trying to say, which are common issues for Parkinson's people.

Patient Name: Robert Smith   Today's Date: 11/2/10

Neurologist: Confidential

Primary Care Physician: Confidential

Please list medications you are currently taking: see attached

Please list your current medical complaints:

Regular exercise has helped. This week I was supposed to be in DC for a park service meeting and had to send someone less qualified, could not handle the stress. I am unable to work 3-4 hours a day. The rest of the day my focus is not great and it takes me longer to do my work. I felt pretty good over the holidays but on Monday at work was bad with tremors. It still takes 3 hours before I can leave work. Yesterday I had an appointment with disability carrier and had to have him come to the house. I was nauseated, slightly dizzy, weepy from stress and shaky.
Last week we were interviewing with the park service and I was shaking extremely bad and had to sit on my arm. When I stood up, my arm was out of control.
I don't know if we were selected.

PRESCRIPTION RENEWAL

The doctor is always asking if I need any new "scripts."

I always tease him by saying, "My subscriptions to *Sports Illustrated, Pro Football Weekly*, and *Wine Spectator* are current, thank you."

"No, your medicine renewals."

Oh. Well, how am I supposed to know that off the top of my head?

After a couple of years of conversations like this, I finally decided to not just sit there like a dummy. The first step is to line up all your pill containers in front of you and make a list of all your medications. Then add columns with how many renewals are left and when they need to be refilled. Now your doctor won't look puzzled. It's all there in black and white!

Medication List
Date: 6/10/15

	Medication (Function)	Quantity	Refills Left	Last Filled	Next Refill
1	Carbidopa-Levodopa Enta (Parkinson's)	90	2	5/30/15	6/20/15
2	Trihexyphenidyl (Parkinson's)	45	0	4/16/15	7/16/15
3	buPROP SR (Antidepressant)	180	1	6/4/15	9/4/15
4	Alprazolam (Anxiety & Stress)	180	4	7/7/15	8/7/15
5	Lisinopril (Blood Pressure)	90	0	6/4/15	9/4/15
6	Hydrochlorothiazide (Blood Pressure)	36	0	6/7/15	9/715
7	Atorvastatin (Cholesterol)	90	0	5/4/15	8/4/15

PARKINSON'S MEDICATIONS

The medication discussion of Parkinson's treatment may seem vague, uninteresting, and like too much medical jargon for most people; but in reality, this is the heart of defense. You will be spending the rest of your life dealing with pills to push Parkinson's back. There will likely be a huge learning curve for both you and your neurologist, since little is known on where to begin treatment and with what medications. It may sound exhausting, but when you are fighting a disease without a cure, there is a lot of trial and error until you find the right medication for your system.

There will be drugs that make you nauseous, and others that will create compulsive behavior traits. It's all in the small print on the medication package where they address side effects that could become your reality. You just do not know which side effects you will experience with each medication. Talk to your neurologist about switching medications if one is not working for you. Don't wait a year, like I did, and suffer more than you need. There is enough to deal with physically and mentally when you're living with Parkinson's, and there's no need to be more overwhelmed trying to make sense of your fight with a chronic disease. Let's not forget—stress, anxiety, and depression will complicate and often make it difficult to ascertain which medication is the culprit in making you feel like crap.

During the initial appointment with my neurologist, we discussed which medication he would prescribe for treating my Parkinson's symptoms, which consisted mainly of tremors and movement disorders.

There are two classes of medication currently used to treat Parkinson's: one is Dopamine Agonist and the other is Levodopa, which is the most common treatment for Parkinson's. After reading several articles regarding Levodopa, it seems to be the most effective drug for treating a wide array of symptoms, ranging from tremors to stiffness to muscle control and balance. Dopamine Agonist is often the first Parkinson's medications given to help with stiffness and muscle control, but for me had more side effects than Levodopa. All of the medications have one goal, and that is to produce dopamine.

For the first several years of treatment for Parkinson's, my medications were based on Dopamine Agonists such as Requip and Mirapex, which are brand-name drugs. The side effects I was experiencing consisted of nausea (it would knock me down for several hours in the morning), vomiting, falling asleep without warning, compulsive behavior traits, increasing tremors, and, to top it off, weight gain. The compulsive behavior issues can range from gambling to alcohol abuse to sexual and drug addictions. Your doctor and caregiver should be on the lookout if any of these issues appear.

The Dopamine Agonist-derived medications were not working for me. If it does not work in the short term, it will not work in the long term. Sad, but true.

The switch to Levodopa-based medication, such as Stalevo, was like night and day. The tremors were significantly reduced, and the nausea, stiffness, and movement disorders subsided, along with compulsive behavior issues. My outlook on life improved, and I started down the path to a positive attitude!

Switching from one medication to another needs to be done gradually, bringing one down and the other up. The drugs may stay in your system for a long period of time while the new prescription takes effect.

Changes in medications are common and often relate to my ever-evolving mental and physical condition. I have found that after a long period of time, many medications lose their effectiveness. Each person's makeup is different. Some people love Mirapex. Others hate it. For me, it was a nightmare. It generated abnormal side effects and compounded the effects of my depression medications.

After several years of trial and error with various combinations, we have found that Stalevo (Levodopa) and Wellbutrin were compatible with my system. Don't be afraid of switching depression medications, as well, as there are a number of them on the market. Prior to Wellbutrin, I was taking Cymbalta, which helped to control my depression slightly but left me with a low libido. It was five years before I settled on Stalevo and Wellbutrin.

If you are looking for the ideal combination, it will probably not happen. You put up with the minor issues that make it bearable. At this point, I am quite satisfied with reaching 75% of normal. The good part of dedication to building a strong offense, which you'll read about in the next chapter, is that I have been able to reduce or eliminate medications, making it easier on my system. It's a whole new world of relief moving forward. Whenever possible, I work with my doctor to consider generics as a suitable substitute to brand-name medications. Your Medicare Supplement D plan emphasizes generics, which helps when you are on a budget. The list of my current medications follows. This list is ever-changing, as my body dictates what it needs. By the time this book is printed, the list will probably be inaccurate, but I want you to see it as a snapshot in time. My goal is that through a powerful Offense, there will eventually be less dependence on pills.

Medication List	
Carbidopa-Levodopa-Enta (Stalevo)	Parkinson's
buPROP SR (Wellbutrin)	Antidepressant
Alprazolam	Anxiety and stress
Lisinopril	Blood pressure
Hydrochlorothiazide	Blood pressure
Atorvastatin	Cholesterol

LATEST PARKINSON'S MEDICATIONS

Rytary

Rytary is a new medication which helps to alleviate the "off" time between doses when the tremors come back as a result of not having sufficient dopamine available. Rytary has essentially the same components as Stalevo, but with an extended release feature that bridges the down time between doses. Impax has a Patient Assistance Program which provides this medication at no cost, as it is a brand name drug with limited or no coverage by the Medicare Supplement D program.

Xadago

Xadago was approved in 2017 by the FDA. It is an add-on medication to Carbidopa-Levodopa, positioned as a once-daily medication to alleviate the "off" time between regular doses. Xadago is in the production phase in the United States; Newron Pharmaceuticals has not set a release date, but it is currently available in several European countries. Xadago is being hailed as the first approved Parkinson's medication in ten years.

ADDITIONAL TREATMENT OPTIONS

Stem Cell Treatment

While searching for information on the difference between Dopamine Agonists and Levodopa, I came across a site on stem cell treatment for Parkinson's, which appears promising. I was surprised and encouraged to discover stem cell treatment is moving forward and is actually being used as an alternative to traditional Parkinson's medication and, most importantly, is working for people now. I have always felt a treatment would come along that would be able to provide a self-healing alternative to traditional medication.

Hope for a cure is so important to those suffering and dealing with Parkinson's on a daily basis. Even if it is years down the road, stay positive in your outlook on life.

Deep Brain Stimulation

I recently attended a presentation on Deep Brain Stimulation for people with Parkinson's disease at a local hospital. There were about forty people in attendance with Parkinson's or MS. The audience was definitely there to learn more about an alternative method of treatment. They presented a video that highlighted how Deep Brain Stimulation was performed. Brain stimulation would definitely help those with advanced Parkinson's. It seems crazy, but the treatment involves drilling a hole in your brain to implant an electrode that will stimulate the brain to make dopamine. They then fish a wire under your skin to a button on your chest, which you push to send a signal that triggers the brain to produce dopamine. I'm not sure I would want to go this route at this stage for dealing with Parkinson's, but it is showing to be an effective option for those with advanced stages of the disease.

MEDICAL HISTORY

Medical Records

Obtain copies of all your medical records from at least the last three to five years. Compare results as often as possible, because it will be one of the first clues that a complication is arising. These clues may offer the opportunity for early intervention. Your medical records are important and should not be set aside for any reason.

Blood Work

It is important to have blood and urine lab work taken on a regular basis during your biannual visit. Many medications can have adverse effects on your body, especially on the liver and kidneys. The test results should hit the mid-point range of the high or low marks. The doctors can then feel comfortable in modifying your medication regime.

PLAYING BY THE LEAGUE RULES AND REGULATIONS

The topics of Social Security, disability, and Medicare are complex. It has taken quite a bit of head scratching to even get a basic understanding of these important topics. The best way to discuss them might be to explain the topics as a series of steps.

When to Stop Work

There will be a point in time when fighting Parkinson's disease and working are not compatible. You will know when your movement issues keep accelerating and the cognitive aspects impact your ability to hold down a job. Once you have taken that step, there is a choice to be made on whether to go on part-time or full-time disability. All of the programs accommodate that choice. For myself, I was pretty far along with Parkinson's symptoms and the difficulty in dealing with day-to-day tasks in an impaired state. The decision was simple: I needed to be on full-time disability. In many cases, working part-time might still be an option. (The paperwork is the same for both.)

Social Security Disability

If you are under the age of 65, you can apply for Social Security disability benefits before reaching the normal age of 66 for Social Security benefits. The parameters are that you expect to be out of work for one full year and that your illness is on the list of impairments. Records and opinion from your doctor will be needed to verify your condition. Once you are approved for disability, Medicare eligibility is available with the disability program. The timeline for approval can be lengthy. To fully understand coverage, speak to a Social Security Advocate, which is offered at no cost. They are best qualified to determine your eligibility.

Social Security

Upon reaching the age of 66, you become eligible for Social Security benefits if you contributed into the program. There are other plans that are similar for teachers, public employees, and other agencies. Working in the private sector, Social Security was part of my retirement income.

Spousal benefits are also available on a 50% basis of the primary participant's benefits. Many people work prior to full retirement age while receiving Social Security, in which case a portion will be deducted from your benefit check. After full retirement there is no restriction on how much you earn. Contact your local social security office for full and complete information.

Health Insurance

Medicare is the program that provides your healthcare coverage under the Social Security umbrella. There are four parts to the Medicare Plan, with distinct providers for each. It is one plan, but you make payment separately to Medicare and your health care provider, which is a private insurance company.

- **PART A:** Covers hospital, skilled nursing facility, home health, and hospice care. This part is paid for under the Medicare program and is deducted from your Social Security benefits.

- **PART B:** Covers doctors, preventive care, medical equipment, hospital outpatient, laboratory tests, x-rays, and mental health care. This part of Medicare is provided by a private health care insurance company. Medicare does not pay Part B; it is the individual who is responsible for payment.

- **PART C:** An alternative plan in lieu of Part B, which is called Medicare Advantage Plans.

- **PART D:** Prescription Drug Coverage, again provided by a private insurance company you pay as part of the Medicare program. Drug coverage costs are regulated for what they pay and what comes out of your pocket.

Disability Income Insurance

Disability income insurance is similar to life insurance, except it provides for income if you are disabled and cannot work. Income benefit payouts can be from three years to lifelong. Premiums will vary accordingly to the number of years designated in the policy. The cost to begin coverage is determined by your age. The policy premium escalates with your age when you start coverage.

COST OF FIGHTING PARKINSON'S

The Parkinson's Team

GENERAL PRACTITIONER: Office visits are generally twice a year, with a co-pay of $50 per visit covered by your primary health care provider for an annual cost of $100. Bloodwork is normally covered by your plan.

NEUROLOGIST: Generally, there are four appointments a year with a co-pay of $50 per visit, or $200 per year.

PSYCHOLOGIST: A therapy session of one hour generally costs $125 with six visits per year over a three year period, or $750 annually. During my most difficult time dealing with the mental and emotional turmoil, sessions every two weeks were necessary to make changes in my life.

ALTERNATIVE THERAPIES: Generally, six appointments a year at $90 to $125 per visit. Annual costs would range from $540 to $750.

Fitness Plan

FITNESS CENTER: Private health clubs can range from $70 to $125 per month, depending the type of facilities offered. Public recreation centers often offer seniors what is called a "Silver Sneakers Program" for about $10 per month. An additional benefit of a recreation center is that they often have a swimming pool and offer water exercise programs for people with Parkinson's or other movement disorders. Exercise classes, including yoga, are usually part of the membership benefits.

PERSONAL TRAINER: A trainer typically costs approximately $65 per 45-minute session once a week for a month for a cost of $260, then biweekly for a cost of $130 a month. The personal trainer costs would be $1,690. The number of sessions per month can be adjusted to your income; once a month would at least make you aware of exercise plans you can do on your own to target your needs. From my experience, weekly personal training sessions are optimal to maintain a mindset that doesn't waiver from the goal that exercise is the most important part of your wellness plan. I realize this is probably the most expensive portion of the plan, but it has the highest value and reward of all the strategies to stay ahead of Parkinson's. I have tried working out on my own program, but there is no substitute for a knowledgeable professional who can work towards specific exercises that will benefit a person with Parkinson's.

Medications

The number of medications prescribed by your general practitioner and neurologist can vary greatly, which affects your monthly cost outlay. The basic medications I take include Parkinson's medications and medications for anxiety, depression, blood pressure, and cholesterol, all of which cost approximately $1,200 annually, or $100 a month. The cost is based on the coverage provided by your primary health care plan for Part D (Medicare coverage). Most medications cost from $3 to $20 per month for generic brands, which lowers your cost significantly versus using brand name medications. One exception is my Parkinson's medication, which is a generic. The cost for the first eight months of the year were $20 per month, then for the remaining four months of the year the out-of-pocket cost jumped to an average of $145 per month upon reaching a plan limit level that provides less coverage. My out-of-pocket medication cost for the past year was $1,200. The costs paid by the Medicare prescription drug coverage (Part D) plan for the year saved me $3,400.

Supplements

The monthly supplement expenditure could run approximately $80 to $120 per month, or $960 to $1,440 annually based on your individual program. I purchase all of my supplements online from Vitacost, the exception being Mucuna Puriens (liquid extract) which is from Banyan Botanicals.

The first three years of implementing the Playbook to turn around my health were the most costly. However, the costs for doctors, health insurance, medications, and supplements are fairly constant. Most health clubs and group fitness classes offer a senior discount with free group fitness classes, which is a substantial reduction in cost. The personal trainer sessions vary from biweekly to once a month, which is a minimum to keep on track. I attend yoga classes three days a week, one day with a personal trainer, and one day following my set program of cardio and general strength building. After three years, I only see the psychologist and alternative therapist on an as-needed basis. I have found that if you ask for a discount or price reduction, people are glad to support your efforts to fight Parkinson's.

HOME SAFETY

As noted at the beginning, we're playing this game at home. Think of this as the work the grounds staff has done setting up the field to best suit our playing style. For that, our corners are proactive and aggressive, playing the man up close and personal—totally in tune with our defensive philosophy of getting the ball back and giving it to our offense.

The crucial concept here is setting up the home to minimize and, better still, totally remove any risk of falling. Falling has a number of unhealthy consequences: injury, including broken bones, with the potential of being unable to exercise and all the attendant issues that raises, including life-threatening respiratory issues; and the emotional and mental toll over the loss of independence and fear of future falls.

Re-Organize Furniture, Rugs, and All Trip-and-Fall Risks

De-clutter. Create relatively wide, straight lines of access to avoid having to dodge around objects to get from A to B. Keep the floor adjacent to walls relatively clear (walls provide a safe haven to lean against). Minimize the use of rugs; there will be times when you shuffle, and you'll absolutely trip and fall on an area rug.

Look out for protruding furniture legs and sharp edges, as the potential to hurt yourself is high. Remember, every time you hurt yourself, the less likely it is that you'll be willing to put yourself in that position again. That is inhibiting and badly affects quality of life.

Grab Bars

Identify critical areas of movement change: changes in direction (corners), transitions from sitting to standing, and steps (hopefully none). Install "grab bars," something to grab ahold of in the event you can't negotiate the change in direction well. Hand/foot/eye (spatial) coordination will become compromised, and at these critical points— changes in direction—the safety of having something to grab ahold of is paramount.

Railings at Stairs

There will likely come a time when stairs are no longer an option. Until that happens, stairs are where you are most vulnerable. Move with extreme caution all the time, every time. It's too late to be careful after you've fallen! At the very least, install and use rails at all stairs. Always stay on the widest part of the steps.

Higher Toilet

Transitioning from sitting to standing can be dangerous when you're struggling with coordination and balance. Medications can sometimes be constipating, and going to the bathroom can be a traumatic experience. Trying to rise from a normal toilet height can be difficult, and in a somewhat compromised state (due to pain or blood pressure changes), you can fall. Reduce the risk of falling by installing a higher toilet and grab bars. If that is not an option, look at a raised toilet seat with handrails.

Shower Bench

Many people fall in the shower. This can be the result of a combination of standing for a relatively long period of time and the effect of the hot water. Plus, with balance and flexibility issues, slipping on the wet surface becomes a constant issue. A simple bench to sit on mitigates against such an eventuality.

Built-Up Utensils

Oftentimes, it becomes difficult to hold and use utensils. Special built-up utensils are available that make eating less of an issue. It's much better, psychologically, to use the utensils than to look with trepidation toward each and every mealtime, wondering what catastrophe will befall you this time!

Clothing and Shoes

Buttons, especially very small buttons, progressively become more difficult to deal with. Shoelaces can also become an issue - not just in the tying, but in the potential for creating the conditions for a fall. Start thinking ahead when buying clothing and choose pieces that use zippers and Velcro.

Touch-Sensitive Lamp Switches

Switches, especially rotatable light switches, become problematic. Consider changing to touch-sensitive switches.

House Access

Access to the house is going to become an issue. Start looking at the options, especially with the potential of needing wheelchair access using a ramp. You should think about any exterior ramp construction providing the ability to move in and out during the winter (with potentially wet and icy conditions), as well as nighttime lighting.

Garden Access

When making changes to outdoor patios, factor in wheelchair access. You don't want to go to all the trouble of creating a wonderful space outdoors and then not be able to use it because you can't get around it while using a walker or wheelchair.

DEFENSE ALONE ISN'T GOING TO DO IT

When I started taking the medications, things just got progressively worse: the tremors, the troubled walking, and the stuttered thinking. Those feelings I had after the doctor handed me the negatives to my MRI—alone, confused, and scared—didn't leave me for years.

Yes, I had family that cared for me, a wonderful wife that wanted to support me, and doctors, but I didn't have anyone who knew what I was going through and could help me from inside. I was completely alone, trying to figure out how to cope with life with Parkinson's, when the inevitable happened.

I was giving a presentation at work. With dozens of eyes upon me, I felt my heart begin to race and my right arm begin to shake.

"Well, I think . . . it's important . . . to . . ." I grabbed my right arm with my left hand and tried to hold it still, but I could barely keep track of my train of thought. "The first thing we need to address is . . . and then . . ." As the tremors accelerated, I leaned toward the conference table, trying to pin my arm down between my chest and the table. "I want to make sure we start it with . . ."

Oh no. There is no hiding it now.

The panic switch had been flipped, and as hard as I tried, I could not manage it. So I did the only thing left to do. I sat on my arm.

It was a federal contract, and the firm had worked hard for it. The stakes were high, the pressure I felt as the leader was beyond what I could handle, and the presentation we were prepping for was scheduled the following day.

"You guys. I have to tell you something. I was diagnosed with Parkinson's disease and I think this is my last presentation on my own."

Silence. The room was thick with uncertainty.

"I need you," I nodded toward my partner, "to run the show, and the rest of you to take on various parts of the presentation. I obviously need to be part of it, but I'm only going to do a small part."

Still silent and wide-eyed, they looked like they were searching inner databases for the appropriate words.

I pushed through the rest of the meeting, and they all pulled themselves together to get the job done.

The next day was virtually the end of my career. I could barely keep the tremors managed during the presentation, and when I went on stage, my arm flailed from my body and up over my head. I was inconsolable for days afterward.

They don't even know the worst of it, I thought as a tear escaped onto my pillow the following day. *But it's only a matter of time before I'm found out. I won't be able to hide all that either.*

It was early in the game, and the defense wasn't enough. I was losing the game. My days of playing defense and hiding were coming to a quick end.

GO ON OFFENSE

"Winning isn't everything . . . It's the only thing."
—VINCE LOMBARDI

L ooking up into the sweaty faces of some of his best defensive players, the coach yells, "We need more than defense today. They're playing hard and keeping us out of the end zone, and it's time for us to change it up on them."

He points down at his tablet and begins to outline the next few plays he wants them to run. It's time to get the ball back and do something with it.

"You got it? It's time to go on the offense. Get that ball back, and let's crush them."

All hands in, the cheer goes up, and they run back out to the field, determined not to lose to this team.

THE INTERVENTION

It was September 2010—the peak and the end of the era.

Our friends, David and Gayla Burnett, had flown in to help me and my wife figure out how to transition out of my career and into disability, and it wasn't long before they began to connect the dots between the credit card bills, the strange phone calls in the middle of the night on family vacations, and my increased isolation, and uncover the compulsive behavior habits that I had been hiding.

That's when David stepped in, with an intensity I had never before witnessed in him.

"Bob, this has to stop. Now. If you don't change, something bad is going to happen to you. You are on the verge of losing everything—your marriage, your family, your self-respect, and any chance at winning against this disease. Enough is enough. This has got to stop."

I hung my head in shame. "I know. But I don't know how to stop it, David."

"Well, I do," he said emphatically. "It's not going to be pleasant or easy, but it's your only chance." His words hung in the air between us for moments before he repeated them, "It's your only chance."

I slowly lifted my gaze, willing myself to get over the embarrassment and listen to my friend, who also happened to be brilliant in his work of helping the body remember how to heal itself.

"I've been working on a protocol for you, Bob."

"David, I'm willing to try anything,"

What he laid out for me was nothing short of a master plan that he had personalized just for me by making it a playbook and using football jargon.

Hope began to stir in my heart as I looked over the document in front of me.

IT'S TIME TO GO ON OFFENSE
David and Gayla Burnett

The typical medical response to a diagnosis of Parkinson's disease is to treat the inevitably worsening symptom constellation with an expanding and increasingly complex regime of protocols and medications.

The underlying sense of the typical treatment convention is that the patient is a *victim* of the progression of the disease and there is little, if anything, that can be done to mitigate the slow but inexorable degradation in quality of life. By its very nature, the approach is defensive—always responding to the next crisis and the onset of an ever-worsening range of debilitating symptoms and dysfunction.

Due to the complex, degenerative, and progressive nature of the condition, there is little credence given to complementary and alternative medical (CAM) options; when they are utilized, they tend to be an ad-hoc "each practitioner looking out for their own turf" approach. The medical community's general lack of knowledge and understanding of CAM options, and fear of interfering with the traditional medical approach, significantly limit the choices available to Parkinson's sufferers. Therefore, the use of CAM typically perpetuates the defensive and reactive approach taken by the traditional medical community.

The typical Parkinson's treatment protocol might consist of 80 to 100 percent traditional medicine and 0 to 20 percent alternative medicine. The outcome of this treatment regime is a steady and progressive worsening of symptoms and loss of quality of life, concurrent with an escalation in treatment protocols until the inevitable happens—the patient succumbs from the complications of Parkinson's. *It doesn't have to be this way!*

What is the Parkinson's Protocol?

The Parkinson's Protocol is a comprehensive, integrated system of lifestyle choices created and optimized for the sole purpose of positively influencing the day-to-day interaction with Parkinson's disease. The protocol provides a broad array of choices that, if followed in part or in whole, significantly:

- Improves day-to-day quality of life

- Provides the opportunity to make positive and informed lifestyle choices

- Slows the progress of the disease

The Parkinson's Protocol does *not* change the underlying medical diagnosis and is *not* a cure for Parkinson's disease.

Foundational Principles

Whatever the current state of the body and regardless of symptoms and dysfunction, with the right input, those symptoms and dysfunctions can be improved. Additionally, the symptoms and dysfunctions do not have to progress along a traditional Parkinson's path. It doesn't have to be this way.

EXERCISE: When exercise is the most important thing in your life, you are exercising just enough. This includes physical exercise (flexibility, balance, and strength) such as yoga, biking, dance, and boxing, and specific brain exercises such as crossword puzzles, Sudoku, or developing new skills in art and music.

SLEEP: Nighttime sleep is critical to enabling the body to recover from, and prepare for more, exercise. Sleep has to be rejuvenating.

NUTRIENTS: You need fuel to sustain more exercise. The body needs nutrients to withstand the increased activity levels and to naturally (innately) heal and restore the physiologic problems it faces. Nutrients include both diet and supplements—particularly foods and supplements that feed the brain.

STRESS: It robs the body of precious physical and energetic resources. Stress contributes to worsening symptoms. Reduce overall stress while improving the management and control of what remains by accentuating positives and minimizing negatives.

YOU ARE WHAT YOU BELIEVE—THE CHOICE IS YOURS. Parkinson's is a diagnosis. Parkinson's is a label. The absolute core belief here is: *If the body can create it (Parkinson's symptoms), then with the right inputs, the body can rebuild itself, in part or in full.*

The *baggage* associated with Parkinson's weighs you down and contributes to a worsening and progressively debilitating condition.

You can be a victim of your diagnosis . . . or you can choose from clearly-defined lifestyle options that positively influence and change the way Parkinson's affects you on a day-to-day basis.

You can take charge of your diagnosis. You can choose to believe something different about Parkinson's and its progression, and then *do something about it.*

Accept:

- Present and future symptoms and dysfunction *do not have to be.*

- There are innumerable lifestyle options and choices, including the choice to be proactive and take the fight to Parkinson's.

- You have the *choice* to leave no stone unturned in the pursuit of improving your quality of life.

Every Day Make Choices Based On:

- What you want to do

- What you can do

- What you can afford to do

- What you actually do

- The knowledge that every choice you make will have some influence on your quality of life

- The reality that you are now, and will continue to always be, a work in progress

While a strong defense takes the ball away from the opposition (Parkinson's), slowing the disease down, a strong offense on the field will score points (improving symptoms and slowing the progression of the disease).

Your Offensive Goal: Score

The goal is to keep the offense on the field and score points, thereby improving or maintaining your quality of life. *"Leave no stone unturned in the pursuit of a quality life."* Make one change at a time. If you make too many changes at once, you won't know what is working or what is causing a problem. Diary everything. Don't rely on your memory! If something (or someone) is not contributing, stop doing it (or sit them). Don't waste time and money. With that being said, if you haven't tried it, you'll never know how much help it may have been.

Key Offensive Players and Coaches
The Quarterback: You

You are the single most important player on the field. In this game, you are the owner and the player. You can't sit on the bench! To play, you need to train. Exercise will keep you mobile, and mobility keeps you from being flattened by the opposition (Parkinson's). More than any one other thing, exercise has the potential to pressure the opposition and control the game. Exercise contributes to a higher-functioning mind and body and improves sleep. It's important that you find someone who can tailor your exercise routines to your condition. Don't waste your time doing what you think is important, only to find it's not optimal. Vary what you do, don't hurt yourself, involve others, and make it *fun*.

Offensive Co-Coordinator Coaches: Doctors, Counselors, and Yoga Therapists

The offensive coordinator is the doctor, counselor, or therapist best able to *identify, coordinate, and manage* the offense. They must be willing to embrace the offensive philosophy of playing the game in the opposition's half. You rarely score points from your end of the field! If you're not playing offense, then you are, by definition, playing defense and ceding the field advantage to the opposing offense! You need a person who recognizes that "time of possession" is an important component in scoring points (quality of life)!

Drill Time: Training and Fitness Program

Total body fitness is the heart and soul of dealing with Parkinson's. The term "exercise" is really too focused. The goal is a fitness program that considers everything from head to toe.

As I started achieving results from my fitness program, the tendency was to overlook the real goal, which is a body that is flexible and balanced. As my body started looking and feeling better, the initial reaction was to start using weights and exercise machines that emphasize muscle mass but decrease flexibility. The exception for including some weight-training to your fitness program is when the body reaches the point of being too lean and starts to lose body mass. A moderate weight-lifting program helps to strengthen the body's structural (bone) system and muscle tone.

It has taken four years to figure out that I want my body to be flexible and trim. Sometimes it takes a while to grasp the concept of total fitness, including the brain. The fitness program for a Parkinson's person is quite different than typical exercise routines. My goal now is a body that is flexible, balanced, coordinated, and lean.

DRILL TIME:
TRAINING AND FITNESS PROGRAM
David and Gayla Burnett

Balance and Core Strengthening
(Pilates, Balance Boards, and Bosu Balls)

Balance, also known as "fall prevention," is critical. Think of it as "poise in the pocket"—no fumbles. Strengthening the core (the bodily region bounded by the abdominal wall, the pelvis, the lower back, and the diaphragm and responsible for its ability to stabilize the body during movement) will help maintain structural integrity, maintain and even improve posture, and contribute to improved balance when standing, transitioning from sitting to standing (a dangerous movement for Parkinson's patients), and walking. It will give you confidence to keep moving. Fear of falling will limit and impede your life, and thereby reduce your quality of life. Pilates concentrates on working the body with a series of floor exercises that emphasizes stretching, rotating, and flexibility movements in a low impact routine.

A bosu ball is a half ball, flat on the bottom and a half moon shape on top, which is spongy and good for balance exercises. Stepping up and down on the ball and pausing when you are on top of the ball is the challenge. As your balance improves, try a series of squats to increase the difficulty. A balance board is the opposite of a bosu ball, with a flat top and rounded bottom where you balance on the board with both feet.

Flexibility and Stretching
(Training Bands and Light Weights)

Second behind balance is flexibility. Think of it as mobility, or "scrambling out of the pocket." Loss of flexibility is the single biggest contributor to pain, discomfort, and the loss of mobility. Your ability to continue to function physically is totally determined by your degree of flexibility. Maintaining flexibility contributes to quality of life. Establish a daily stretching routine of at least 30 minutes. Training bands are elastic in nature and are used to stretch various muscle groups with the goal to lengthen them to improve flexibility. Parkinson's continually constricts your muscles and limits your mobility. Light weights are used for adding resistance in exercises, but not bodybuilding.

Mind-Body Connection
(Tai Chi and Yoga)

The mind-body connection is central to improving your physical and mental health. The best way to do that is with Tai Chi or yoga. It reduces stress, contributes to both flexibility and strength, improves breathing, creates a heightened level of body awareness, and creates an inner strength and resiliency. It also improves sleep. Both Tai Chi and yoga emphasize coordinated movements that require the brain to send a series of messages to various parts of the body to perform an exercise. This helps to reinforce the mind-body connection. Yoga is a total-body and mind workout that combines poses with deep breathing and mediation. Tai Chi is similar to yoga, with poses that are more soft martial arts style but spiritual in nature.

Going into my first full yoga session, I looked around at the class, which consisted mostly of women and just a couple of men. The initial thought was that I would have no problem keeping up with this group. Boy, was I ever wrong! The women were flexible and strong. The interesting part was no one judged me on my ability to complete a pose. I was like a stick figure. The yoga class was really challenging and showed me how far I needed to go if I was going to keep up with Parkinson's determination to immobilize me. I finally understood how hard it was to bend like a pretzel. The yoga trainer encouraged me to continue practicing the various poses on my own. They gave me hope that I could improve my flexibility, balance, and coordination.

Brain Strength
(Crosswords, Sudoku, and Brain Games)

And you thought exercise was only of the physical variety! Think how you will make plays if you don't spend time learning the playbook and being able to read the defense. Ultimately, this game is all about your brain—*use it or lose it*! You need to exercise the brain as much as, if not more than, you do physical activity. Minimize brainless activities. Constantly challenge the brain to maintain its abilities and coordination. If you see a skill becoming impaired, find a brain exercise to re-establish it. Learn new things: take up art or music, become a writer, do anything to activate the brain and keep it busy. Brain games force the mind to think and come up with solutions, as opposed to mindless activities such as watching television.

VARIETY IS KEY

It's important to incorporate as many different activities into your overall exercise regime as possible. They add variety, brain challenge, coordination, and a sense of accomplishment. They are also physically more demanding than those listed earlier.

- Walking, jogging and running outdoors
- Walking on a treadmill with varied speed control
- Biking (on a stationary bike)
- Strength training with weights
- Swimming
- Rock wall climbing (indoors)
- Informal sports such as flag football, soccer, handball, softball, baseball, golf, or tennis

FITNESS

Beginning an exercise program is a significant step in your fight against Parkinson's and should be done in progressive stages. I would highly recommend starting your exercise program under the direction of a yoga therapist or fitness trainer to first evaluate your current physical condition and then guide you through your practice. It makes sense to start at a level that can gradually show improvement. Expecting quick results by overdoing your capabilities will only lead to injuries that will set you back in your efforts to be fit and flexible. Many fitness clubs and recreation centers offer group classes, which are a great way to start your exercise program, as they have classes geared to many levels, from beginner to advanced. Each person is at a different stage in their Parkinson's progress, and you need to be realistic in your expectations. It has taken me many years of steady progression to reach some of the goals set each year. Don't overdo it in the beginning. As they say, slow and steady wins the game.

MORE ON FITNESS

By Alana Foeller
(Yoga Therapist, Ayurveda Practitioner, and Registered Nurse)

I began working with Bob as his personal trainer in 2005, prior to the onset of his Parkinson's symptoms. Our focus originally was strength and cardiovascular training for overall fitness and health. After Bob's diagnosis with Parkinson's, it was apparent that we needed to shift gears and address his symptoms (muscle rigidity, poor balance and coordination, and tremors worsened by stress), so we moved to a yoga therapy program, which focused on flexibility, balance, postural improvement, breathing, and relaxation. Bob continued to do light cardio on his own on a weekly basis, and he and I have met twice a week for therapeutic yoga sessions. I was surprised by how well Bob responded to the challenging and unfamiliar practice of yoga. In my opinion, this was a major transition in Bob's path to healing. This journey was an experiment for both Bob and me. As a Certified Ayurveda Practitioner and Yoga Therapist, I had never worked with anyone with Parkinson's before.

From an Ayurvedic perspective, Parkinson's is an imbalance of VATA Dosha, which governs the elements of air and space. When these elements are out of balance, they manifest as anxiety, restlessness, rigidity, variability of digestion, dryness, shakiness or tremors, and emotional instability, to name a few. In Ayurveda, lifestyle changes, proper nutrition, herbal remedies, and yoga are a few of the modalities used to address such imbalances. In Bob's case, the goal was to get him "grounded;" to calm the over-excitable nervous system and address the stiffness and tremors. Nutritional and herbal therapies were only minor players in his care plan, as he was already on many medications, and both Bob and I agreed it best not to put more into the mix to complicate his already overwhelming regimen. I did advise Bob to do regular *Abhyangha* (therapeutic oil massage), which he reports helps calm him overall, but yoga therapy has really been the most effective modality in the management of his Parkinson's.

When we first began yoga, Bob had a tremor (despite the medications he was taking), and his balance was not great. I noticed right away that his usual pattern of breathing was labored and irregular. Rather than taking slow and even breaths, he seemed to breathe using muscles other than the diaphragm—at times even gasping for air. The beauty of yoga is that it is called a practice. You are not to compare yourself to others. You simply take set postures and work to adapt them to your unique body.

In Bob's case, we began very simply with the "Joint Freeing Series," created by Makunda Stiles. These simple postures did wonders for Bob. After regular practice, he had made leaps of progress in functional range of motion and improved posture. We then added standing and balancing poses, as well as chest openers to stretch the tight muscles on the front of his body. He initially had a minor hunch in his upper spine; his shoulders rolled forward and his head jutted forward. Almost all the muscles in his chest were tight and rigid. Since he began regular yoga practice, I've been with him on several occasions where people have exclaimed how much his posture has improved. He stands taller, appears more confident and relaxed, has no tremor, breathes slower and deeper, and moves in a much more functional way.

Possibly the most powerful aspects of the practice of yoga are the ones that go unnoticed by the untrained eye. Through regular practice of meditation, pranayama (breathing), and relaxation, Bob now has a whole toolbox of ways to cope with stress and calm his mind. Initially, Bob complained of anxiety and sleep disruption, and I'm happy to say these areas have improved in his life. Stress will continue to be a huge player in the progression of Parkinson's, so management of stress is key to keeping it manageable and halting progression.

Over the years I have known Bob, I can say that I've learned more from him than he has from me. I've seen him at his highs and his lows. I know the struggle this has been for him, as well as the determination and dedication that he demonstrates daily to beat a disease he was told could take over his life, rendering him disabled. Bob rarely steps down from a challenge. His courage has been his strength in fighting off Parkinson's disease. He has taken his yoga and exercise program to the next level and surprised everyone, including himself, by participating in a 30-plus-mile bike ride to raise money for Parkinson's. Bob has shown me that if you have a goal worth achieving, you never give up!

A TYPICAL TRAINING DAY

A Typical Training Day	
Morning	• Begin the day with breath work and short meditation to start your day, along with stretching to loosen up the body (5–10 minutes). • Take medications and supplements at the required time. • If not exercising at the gym or doing yoga outside of the house, substitute a home yoga routine for 20–30 minutes.
Afternoon	• On days that involve yoga classes, (generally four days a week), begin or end with 20–30 minutes of cardio, which can be the treadmill or the bike. If you go to the gym on non-yoga days, emphasize cardio, pulling movements (such as rows, lat pulls, and hamstring curls), and balance (such as bosu ball or step-ups), and always end with stretching. • Take medications and supplements at the required time. • Lunch is the largest meal of the day (dinner is the smallest). • After meals, take a short walk for 5 minutes or so, to help digestion. • Aim to eat and sleep at the same time each day. **Do the "Joint Freeing Series" by Mukunda Stiles 3–5 days per week. This will keep you flexible. Learn more at www.yogatherapycenter.org.
Evening	• Have a light dinner no later than 2 hours before going to bed. • Take a short walk after dinner. •Take medications at the required time. • End day with journaling, relaxation, meditation, breathing, or savasana.

Yoga Practice

There are several tools and props that we use on a regular basis in most yoga sessions. Usually, the gym provides the accessories for the group yoga classes, but over time you will want your own equipment, both for cleanliness reasons and for practicing at home. It is important to buy quality equipment since you will be using them regularly. The most common items are:

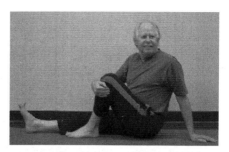

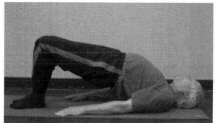

- a yoga mat with a carry case
- a strap for stretching poses to get the most out of the pose
- several sizes of blocks
- a foam roller
- small weight dumbbells
- squeeze hand balls
- toe socks

Your local sporting goods store will likely carry all the equipment you will need, but the yoga supplies and clothing can also be purchased on the Internet if you prefer. The added benefit of having your own equipment means you have become a regular.

At my first yoga class, the terms the yoga instructor used were in a language that was totally unknown to me. It took several months before I figured it out. The good news is that yoga classes follow a slow, flowing rhythm from one pose to another. They might call out "plank" and you look around for a board, but they are saying to get in a push-up position, and then "down dog" where your butt goes up in the air in an inverted "V" shape. Another one is when you end a class with "savasana," which means you get to lay on your back and chill out.

After a while, I bought a couple of books to read about this new yoga practice that I still use to this day. Yoga practice fits so well for the Parkinson's body, from meditation for clearing your mind to stretching and flexibility to strengthening your core to living a healthy life with a happier state of mind. Some of the resources I picked up at the local bookstore to learn about this new form of exercise are the *Yoga Journal Magazine*, *Kundalini Yoga* by Shakta Kaur Khalsa, and *Ten-Minute Yoga for Flexibility and Focus* by Christina Brown.

There are three basic exercise programs that have been specifically tailored for my yoga practice; I have included them in the Resources section at the end of this book, as they might be of some help to your trainer as you start out on the path to fitness. I have also included photos and descriptions for many of the typical poses so you can get an idea of what to expect in a yoga class.

My wife always asks me, "How was yoga class today?" and often I say, "Boy, she wanted us to do the pretzel pose today and I still can't do it. Maybe someday, with more practice, I can get there."

NUTRITION:
YOUR WIDE RECEIVERS
David and Gayla Burnett

Without great wide receivers, your game becomes one-dimensional; you'll spend a lot of time playing defense. You typically don't score many points on defense! Fighting Parkinson's is a demanding task. It takes energy in many different forms. For the body to produce the energy you need to play the game at the highest level, you need to give it plenty of fuel.

Fuel is not just about food (calories). It's really all about the *nutrients* obtained from food. The quantity and quality of nutrients in our regular diet typically do not come close to providing a nutrient-dense foundation for the body and brain to build on. Therefore, we have to do two things: (1) focus on identifying nutrient-rich food to eat, and (2) minimize the bad foods (those with little or no nutrient value) and chemicals that require the body to expend precious energy and resources to process. It's also very important to spread the meals throughout the day. It's unhelpful for the body to be scavenging around (inside itself) looking for nutrients to keep the processes going. Your car doesn't run well if you have a blocked fuel filter—it runs in fits and starts. That's what your body does if you're not eating at least small amounts of balanced, nutrient-rich food every few hours.

Increase Vegetables and Fruits

As a general principle, significantly increase the variety and amount of fruits and vegetables that you consume. While raw has its place, where possible, lightly cooked works best. Try to minimize the use of the microwave when cooking vegetables. Find ways to snack on fruits and vegetables throughout the day.

Identify and Focus on Brain-Friendly Foods

Get alongside a nutritionist familiar with the opposing team (Parkinson's) and identify foods that are considered "brain-friendly." Make sure to incorporate these foods in significant quantities throughout your diet. Brain-friendly foods include spinach, nuts, beets, lentils, and oats, to mention a few. There are many sites on the Internet for additional choices.

Reduce or Eliminate Sugar

They don't call it "White Death" for nothing! Nutritionally speaking, sugar is like the wide receivers' worst nightmare—the dreaded dropped ball or missed catch. You don't score points on offense if the wide receivers keep dropping the ball! Sugar has no purpose other than to change and enhance taste. Find another way to achieve the same purpose by replacing sugar with agave or honey. Also look out for carbohydrates, typically white in color, that turn to sugar in the body. These can include noodles, certain breads, and rice. The body has to expend (waste) precious energy to process these foods. A few common foods to avoid would be candy, some cereals, ice cream, jam/jelly, doughnuts, and pie.

Cut Out Artificial Sweeteners

Artificial sweeteners are as bad as, if not worse than, sugar. These are *toxic chemicals*. Don't put them in your body! The most common artificial sweeteners are Sweet'N Low, Equal, and Splenda. Many beverages, such as tea and soda, also include pre-sweeteners.

Eat the Right Protein

The body needs protein. The open, unanswered question is how much protein do we need, and from what source? Obviously, drug-free and hormone-free protein is best. There are also other protein sources to consider. Soy or white rice is not encouraged, due to the way it is chemically processed. Hemp is another such example. Some research also identifies problems with the timing of protein consumption and interference with the effectiveness of medications. As with all things, you should research that more, as it may be critical. A variety of fish, poultry, meat, cheese, nuts, and beans are acceptable forms of protein. Those that follow a vegan or vegetarian diet have many options to include protein as part of their nutrition plan. Power bars or similar energy products are an option, but be sure to review the ingredients to know what you are consuming.

Reduce Alcohol Consumption

Fundamentally, you can't run routes and catch balls if you've been drinking. That's not to say that you will be penalized after touchdown celebrations. Just do not engage in excessive celebrations and over-exuberance. Remember that alcohol is a *toxin*; it kills brain cells and turns to sugar in the body. Drinking while taking certain medications is dangerous and potentially negates the effectiveness of medications and other things that you are working so hard to achieve. You will pay a price every time you drink. You may be willing to pay that price, and that's okay, but know you are paying a price and setting the offense back. Hard liquor is worse, and should be consumed with caution.

NUTRITION CHART

A balanced diet is important in providing your body with the fuel for maintaining the strength necessary to deal with Parkinson's. The stronger the body, the easier it will be. Keeping a nutrition journal for a week is one approach to evaluating your diet. A simple chart of your food intake over a week will give you a better idea of what it takes for a balanced diet.

Everyone is busy in one way or another. Our family's approach is a set routine; Monday is fish, Tuesday is chicken, Wednesday is pork, Thursday is bison burgers, Friday is pot luck (leftovers), Saturday is chicken again, and Sunday is steak. Variety in how you prepare meals can keep it from feeling routine and boring. For those following a vegan or vegetarian diet, the approach is the same. Simplify your life where possible!

Bob's Example Daily Nutrition Chart

Day #1 Date: January 23, Monday Weight: 156	
Morning Meal Time: 8:00 dried granola, milk, banana, apricots	Water # of ounces today? 60 oz.
Snack Meal Time: 10:00 two slices of pizza	Any additional beverages? glass of white wine
Lunch Meal Time: 2:00 chicken thighs, chips & salsa	What Added Fats? pizza & cheese
Snack Meal Time: 3:00 blueberries, apple	Condiments? pasta sauce & salsa
Dinner Meal Time: 7:00 grilled pork tenderloin, broccoli & pasta	Exercise Type? yoga, stationary bike, treadmill
Snack Meal Time: 9:00 fruit & nuts	Duration of Exercise: 1.5 hrs
What time did you go to bed last night? 11 pm	
What time did you wake up this morning? 7:30 am	
How was your sleep quality? Sound or Restless? Restless	
Did you wake up during the night? once pee, water before bedtime	
Did you wake up feeling refreshed? no, marginal	
Are you sore from your exercise? yes, legs were tired	
Overall energy for the day: good	
Any cravings today? chocolate chip ice cream	

What I learned from the diet chart…

- It has been four years since filling out the diet chart, and the noticeable lifestyle changes over that short period of time have been dramatic.

- Sleep is one of the most important factors on the daily chart, and impacts the day from the moment I get up to when I go to bed. Unbroken nighttime sleep is vitally important. The body restores and recuperates at night, not during daytime naps. If you are not sleeping well and/or waking up un-refreshed in the morning, do something about it. Before going to bed, I take melatonin as a natural sleep aid. If that does not work, then prescription alternatives are better than lack of sleep.

- Consuming too much alcohol triggers a whole bunch of problems, starting with a restless night's sleep. I end up sleeping in, which condenses my nutrition cycle and ability to space out my medications and supplements, all of which contribute to a rough day. It is no wonder I feel like crap until I get enough food in me. Reducing the amount of wine to one glass has made a big difference. The change gives me a full restful eight hours of sleep, with no alcohol after 9 pm, only a glass of water. Now I only get up once a night, which helps me start the day feeling refreshed. I now have fifteen hours of waking time versus the twelve hours. This really helps my outlook.

- **MEALS:** The breakfast was okay, but I needed some protein to last until noon. Pizza shortly afterwards does not cut it as a good diet. The rest of the meals were okay, although the time gets pushed later into the evening. Also, chocolate late at night can keep me up later than I realized. Medication can cause continual problems with constipation; a healthy diet can reduce this issue. Preferably, use natural options first such as fresh and dried fruit, beets, green vegetables, prune juice, etc. If the diet adjustments are not working, then a stool softener may help.

- **EXERCISE:** Even on the weekends, some form of exercise is important. Doing home chores does not cut it. I like to go for a one-mile walk, which takes very little away from the rest of my day.

- **WATER INTAKE:** This is hard to keep track of daily, but without enough water intake, my head can hurt and would make me feel sluggish.

- **MEDICATIONS:** The weekend is an ideal time for organizing a two-week supply of pills in those neat little containers with each day labeled. Just another thing I do not have to think about during my busy weeks.

- **LENGTH OF THE DAY:** It is amazing what an extra three hours does to my daily routine. I have less stress and anxiety because I'm not rushing around at the last minute trying to get all of my medications and supplements down. Taking all that stuff in such a short time can upset my system, making me dizzy, lightheaded, and generally off-kilter.

The blank Nutrition Chart below will get you started in understanding your optimal diet and daily activities, which hopefully will be a benefit to your Parkinson's routine.

Day #1 Date:	Weight:
Morning Meal Time:	Water # of ounces today?
Snack Meal Time:	Any additional beverages?
Lunch Meal Time:	What Added Fats?
Snack Meal Time:	Condiments?
Dinner Meal Time:	Exercise Type?
Snack Meal Time:	Duration of Exercise:
What time did you go to bed last night?	
What time did you wake up this morning?	
How was your sleep quality? Sound or Restless?	
Did you wake up during the night?	
Did you wake up feeling refreshed?	
Are you sore from your exercise?	
Overall energy for the day:	
Any cravings today?	

SUPPLEMENTATION: YOUR OFFENSIVE LINE
David and Gayla Burnett

The foundation of a good offense is a great offensive line. If the offensive line leaks like a sieve and can't protect the quarterback (you), you'll very quickly be playing defense and that's not part of the game plan! The body, and especially the brain, need fuel. A body and brain that are not functioning properly needs even more fuel to function effectively. While we would like to think we can get all the necessary fuel from our diet, the reality is typically the opposite. While much of the supplement market is poor in quality and bioavailability (meaning the body can't process it), there are supplements that the body *can* utilize. The best products typically will not be found at your local grocery store, but online with companies that specialize in supplements.

Green Vibrance

Most multivitamin products are created in a lab using chemical ingredients. The body has to expend resources to process these products. Many come in pill form and are difficult for the body to process. Vibrance is made from raw food and the powder form converts to a liquid, the most body-friendly form. Vibrance will give you all the nutrients you need in a form that is easily useable for your body.

CoQ10 (Ubiquinol)

Numerous studies (opposition scouting reports) have shown a relationship between low levels of CoQ10 and Parkinson's. Some studies show supplementing with CoQ10 has a direct positive influence on your symptoms. CoQ10 is a powerful antioxidant that is critical to body and brain function. If you have been on statin drugs forever, they are known to leach CoQ10 from your body. CoQ10 should be taken from the time you start using cholesterol medication.

Supplements for Brain Support

There is considerable evidence that certain helpful chemicals support brain function and activity. It is also clear that it is very difficult, if not impossible, to get these critical chemicals from our food. Therefore, it is vitally important to supplement with these chemicals on a daily basis.

L-Theanine

L-Theanine is an amino acid that, among other things, stimulates the production of dopamine in the brain. It also reduces stress on the brain and helps you keep focus and attention.

Phosphatidylserine (PS)

This is a phospholipid (a type of healthy fat) found throughout the body, with the highest concentrations in the brain. Preliminary studies have shown PS has a positive effect on brain function, with the potential of inhibiting brain deterioration as we age.

Glutathione

Produced within the body as a result of cellular function, Glutathione is absolutely crucial to effective functioning of many body systems, including the immune and nervous systems. It can be supplemented, but is difficult to get through the digestive process into the body. Glutathione the potential to be a game-changer if we can find a way to effectively get it into the body.

Vitamin D3

Vitamin D3 is absolutely vital to the effective functioning of the immune and nervous systems, but is often chronically depleted in people in this country. Check your levels of vitamin D3 with a simple blood test, and if it is not optimal, supplement it. Make sure the supplement is D3, not just vitamin D.

Vitamin B (Complex)

This is another absolutely vital ingredient to having the body function optimally, but is also often chronically depleted. Again, check your levels with a simple blood test and supplement it if your levels are not optimal.

Creatine

Creatine is an amino acid responsible for providing energy in the muscles. Keeping muscles healthy and energized will contribute significantly to your ability to exercise and stay flexible. As described earlier, your ability to exercise is the single most important factor in your ability to stay on offense.

Magnesium

Magnesium is central to hundreds of internal chemical processes and reactions. It has significant influence on the nervous system and muscles and has positive influence on sleep, but is often chronically depleted.

Essential Fatty Acids (EFA)

When dealing with an illness, one of the most important factors is minimizing collateral damage. When the body is not functioning properly, it knows it; and it prioritizes its internal processes and reactions to provide resources to the area in most need.

This has a cascade effect on the rest of the body, drawing much-needed resources away and creating a negative cascade effect. Essential fatty acids can help mitigate this process. There are different types, and you need to identify those most beneficial to your situation.

Proteolytic Enzymes

Similar in nature to the essential fatty acids described above, photolytic enzymes provide the body with additional resources (in quantities that cannot be obtained through diet alone) to optimize body function and prevent collateral damage.

Hormones (Adrenal Thyroid)

Hormones play a significant role in the efficient and effective functioning of the body. The consequences of them being out of balance can be catastrophic. You may well have experienced some issues already. Still, the changes your body is going through because of the nature of the game, and the changes you will be making, will all place added burden on the pituitary, adrenal, and thyroid glands. It's vital to keep on top of the functioning of these organs. When you have your blood work tested, remember that *normal* readings are not an option—all must be in the *optimal* range.

SUPPLEMENTS LIST

The supplements listed below were developed for my particular health condition and are not suitable for everyone. Consult with your health advisor regarding your specific condition and needs.

These supplements are composed of natural ingredients, serve many functions, and should be taken only for specific health conditions. Some of the supplements can conflict with Parkinson's medications, so noted below are supplements that I used but changed as my medications changed. Everyone reacts differently to supplements, and what works for one might not work for another. It is a full-time job managing your medications and supplements. Even with my team of experts, it still rests on my shoulders to manage a health and fitness plan.

Supplements	Function
Green Vibrance	Nutrient-dense vitamin
Vitamin B Complex	Vitamin supplement
Vitamin D-3	Vitamin supplement
CoQ10	Cellular metabolism
Creatine	Muscle repair and energy
Phosphatidylserine	Memory enhancer
DMAE	Memory enhancer**
L-Theanine	Brain focus and relaxation
L-Tyrosine	Depression *
Mucuna Pruriens (liquid extract)	Natural source of levodopa (L-dopa)**
Melatonin	Sleep aid
Magnesium	Reduce Stress and relaxation
NADH	Energy boost, stamina, and mental clarity

*Can conflict with depression medications; seek medical approval before use
** Can conflict with Parkinson's medications; seek medical approval before use

Most supplements are available online from companies that carry quality products and are generally a fresher product. My preference for purchasing supplements is Vitacost, with the exception of Mucuna, which is sold by Bayan Botanicals. Your grocery store is not the place to buy supplements; the exception would be stores that specialize in natural products.

ALTERNATIVE TREATMENTS

There are two alternatives worth exploring: Mucuna and marijuana. Further research should be done before incorporating them into your treatment plan. With any program, begin with small dosages so you can ascertain the compatibility with your personal situation.

Mucuna Treatment for Parkinson's

Another Parkinson's treatment being explored is Mucuna, which is an herbal composition. The seed powder of the leguminous plant, Mucuna, has been used as treatment in traditional Ayurveda medicine for Parkinson's disease. Since the FDA has not approved Mucuna, the medical community cannot prescribe this as a treatment strategy, and the decision to use an alternative medicine is up to the individual.

Marijuana for Parkinson's

There is increasing use of marijuana as an aid to help reduce tremors. Research and case studies are coming to light showing marijuana being used as an alternative to Parkinson's medications. I have not tried marijuana as part of my program, but will look at its use when my Parkinson's pills' effectiveness wears off between doses.

COMPLEMENTARY AND ALTERNATIVE THERAPIES
David and Gayla Burnett

Complementary Therapies: Your Tight Ends

A great tight end has the potential to be a game-changer. They open the defense up, creating opportunities for others, while at the same time offering the potential to make significant contributions in their own right. A good one is a "keeper."

Each therapist listed below is a specialist. Find ones who understand this particular type of game and are willing to integrate seamlessly into your game plan. When the time is right, they will each contribute their unique abilities to your game.

PHYSICAL THERAPY: A physical therapist will help with improving your mobility, which is essential for those with Parkinson's.

OCCUPATIONAL HEALTH THERAPY: Occupational health therapy is the use of assessment and treatment to develop, recover, or maintain the daily living and work skills of people with physical, mental, or cognitive disorders.

SPEECH THERAPY: One of the ongoing issues with Parkinson's is speaking softly. When people keep asking you to speak louder because they have trouble understanding you, seek help from this specialist.

Alternative Therapies: Your Running Backs

Team effort is the key to the success of this game plan. Your running backs are crucial offensive weapons. Gaining ground, eating up the clock, keeping the offense on the field, and putting enormous pressure on the opponent's defense is the best approach. With the highest-functioning quarterback in the league, star wide receivers, and running behind the most awesome and effective offensive line, your running backs are your best alternative attacking weapon. Use them aggressively and often. Establish the "run," and the other options become more effective. Many of the play options below work with the body, stimulating it to heal itself and optimize its function.

Bowen Therapy

Bowen therapy is the product of Tom Bowen, an Australian who created and practiced the technique from the mid-1950s until his death in 1982. Tom Bowen's work has been carried forward by practitioners who observed him at work.

Within the context of the Parkinson's environment, Bowen therapy is an *invaluable* resource because it effectively works at so many different levels in the body.

Most importantly, Bowen stimulates the body to undertake a complete review of all its systems and functionality and, where possible, initiates restorative and healing processes. Many symptoms just disappear. However, ongoing treatments are needed to combat changes brought about by the degenerative and progressive nature of the disease.

Bowen therapy is the most efficient and successful "structural integrator" in body work. By straightening and aligning the structure, Bowen helps create the foundation for balance and normal movement. In addition, Bowen effectively works the wrists, hands, ankles, and feet.

Some Bowen practitioners have integrated other complementary non-massage neurologic techniques into their Bowen work. Many of these techniques piggy-back off of the underlying therapeutic action of Bowen and are, therefore, more effective than if done alone. They become additive to the effects of Bowen, which inherently stimulates its own strong neurologic effect.

Bowen therapy practice centers on healing the whole body in totality. It is a cross-fiber gently manipulative (muscle-rolling) technique that initiates an immediate and powerful healing influence on the body. Physical changes often take place, and structural irregularities can resolve right on the table without manipulation or adjustment. The body simply "adjusts" itself.

The mechanism of action would appear to be twofold:

- Vibratory (frequency) from the muscle squeezing out from under the rolling movement, stimulating the brain and central nervous system to look for irregularity, thereby triggering a restorative process.

- Pauses (touching breaks) between the movements, allowing the body to assimilate the signal (vibration—frequency—message) and initiate some restorative reaction before the next movement begins. This concept of a definitive pause between movements is rare in bodywork and contrasts considerably from massage, where the therapist's hands are always in contact with, and stimulating, the body.

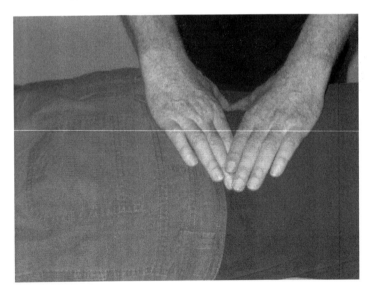

Back

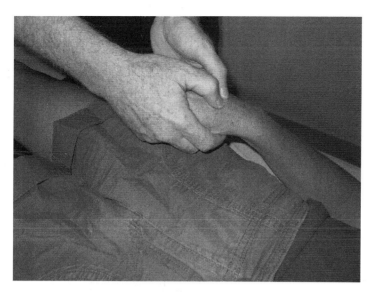

Wrist

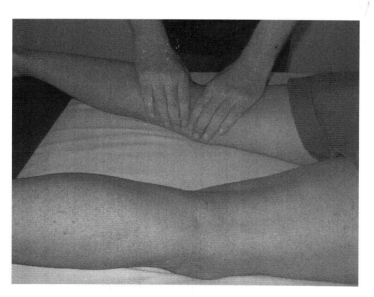

Knee

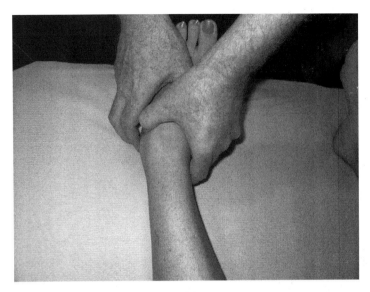

Ankle

Bowen therapy is a whole-body technique, typically performed over clothing. Although there are no specific relaxation movements, most participants experience a deep sense of relaxation during and after a treatment. Bowen works in harmony with the body's restorative and innate healing processes and doesn't impose or force change. There are no adjustments or structural manipulations similar to those found in chiropractic or osteopathic techniques, and Bowen is not massage.

The body typically continues to evolve (improve) in the 72 hours following a treatment before settling into a new and improved state. Follow-up treatments are normally a week apart, where further advances in restoration are made and the pattern of change continues.

Many conditions, including long-standing, chronic structural conditions, resolve in four or fewer treatments, and characteristically, there is no requirement for ongoing maintenance.

MY FIRST BOWEN THERAPY SESSION

I was accustomed to a typical spa massage setting that is tactile, with a masseuse using their hands to loosen muscles and release the knots and tightness held in the body. The massage environment is dimly lit, warm, and cozy, with soothing oil-covered hands that glide over your body in an almost sensual manner with only a towel covering private areas.

"Do I take off my shirt and pants for the Bowen session?" I asked David when he walked into the room.

"No, not at all. I can work through your clothes." He smiled.

David started by aligning my spine, followed by my hips and shoulders. He did these short sequences of moves, and then left the room.

He must have to go to the bathroom, I thought.

He came back, checked his work, and then did a few more moves before leaving the room again.

Gee, he must have a very small bladder.

After the third time, I decided to ask, "Why do you only do a few moves and then leave for a few minutes? Do you have a tiny bladder?"

David laughed out loud before answering, "No. See, with these sequences, I am giving your body the information it needs in order to do the work itself. I'm not pushing anything back into place or realigning your spine; it's *your body* doing the work."

"Wow. That's amazing." I laid there, noticing energy moving through my arms and legs, though all he had touched was my back.

When David finished, he was sweating and had a towel around his neck. My body felt normal, but I was giving off so much energy that the room temperature felt ten degrees warmer to anyone else.

"I'm going for a quick walk to get rid of some of the energy absorbed while you rest for a few minutes," David said. I did not know if it was voodoo or what, but David now had a road map to start my self-healing process on specific parts of my body.

Bowen treatment has enabled me to move forward with a fitness program that is geared to keep Parkinson's on the defense. When I weighed 182 pounds on a 5'6" frame that was out of shape, the thought was I could go to the gym and automatically be on the road to fitness. Boy, was I wrong! When our body is out of alignment, we tend to overcompensate, which leads to sore and strained muscles that are a setback in going to the gym on a regular basis. Being out of alignment means less time for your exercise routines, which is a real roadblock for those with Parkinson's.

My initial experience in 2011 with Bowen treatment was eye-opening and profound. In the early years, the effects of Parkinson's were compounding. As I tried to offset the rigidity from the disease with an irregular exercise program, I was not making headway. The more I tried, the more setbacks from injuring myself were making it difficult to maintain a regular schedule of exercise. After the initial Bowen treatments, my body alignment was improving. The Bowen treatments provided the foundation for improving my fitness level. My yoga therapist was then able to build upon my newfound fitness incrementally. I did not realize it at first, but my trainer was able to start a program of exercise that was geared to making me fit. The most powerful aspect of Bowen is how it helped to stabilize my frame in a self-healing manner.

Bowen treatments need to be reinforced periodically since the body is constantly changing due to Parkinson's. As an example, after a long vacation with considerable walking, my right hip was out of alignment. The pain was getting worse, even when I returned home. Walking around the house and taking it easy did not alleviate the problem. Within two Bowen sessions, the pain was gone and I was able to get back to my exercise routine.

SCENAR TECHNOLOGY
David and Gayla Burnett

The long name for this device is Self-Controlled Energetic Neuro-Adaptive Regulator, also known as SCENAR.

SCENAR was originally developed for the Soviet space program in the late 1970's to heal injuries during flight. It was approved by the USSR Medical Council (the Soviet equivalent of the FDA) in 1986 for use in the Soviet medical system.

SCENAR is a highly sophisticated, non-invasive, battery operated, handheld biofeedback device. SCENAR uses *electro-therapy activation* (radio waves) which stimulates a chemical (neuro-peptide) reaction in the Central Nervous System (CNS).

SCENAR "interacts" with the body in real time, dynamically adjusting its output signal(s) in response to the body's evolving reactions. SCENAR stimulates pathologic change in the body by mimicking the body's own endogenous-bioelectric regulatory communications. In other words, SCENAR "talks" to the body using the body's own language, and the body doesn't identify that the stimuli is external.

A comprehensive array of protocols and device settings orient the treatments geographically in the body—locally into specific 'trauma' areas (injury or post-operative sites) or regionally to address systemic issues throughout the body.

SCENAR has been used predominantly by practitioners in Western Europe and the UK. Similarly, in the United States, SCENAR is primarily used by chiropractors, physical therapists, and naturopaths. Inherent in the general treatment protocols, SCENAR will also stimulate the body to restore and maintain balance within all of its systems.

Specifically, SCENAR will positively influence the localized musculoskeletal issues associated with rigidity and joint articulation in the hands and feet. One aspect critical to maintaining quality of life in those with Parkinson's is confidence in the ability to walk. SCENAR provides a number of different protocols and device settings to ensure and maintain full functionality of the ankles and feet. These same techniques can be used on the wrists and hands.

SCENAR has an integral role to play in the treatment and management of Parkinson's disease.

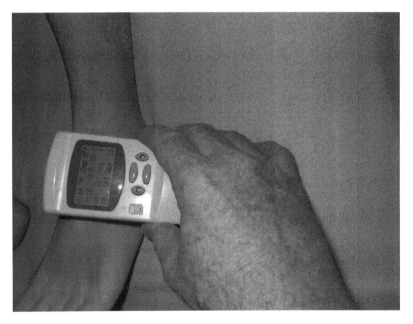

Ankle

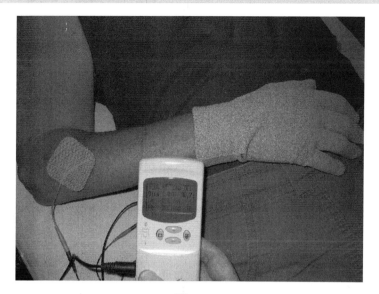

Glove

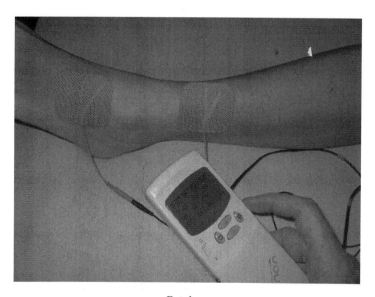

Patches

MY EXPERIENCE WITH SCENAR

"At our Bowen session, I remained dressed. Is it the same for a SCENAR treatment?" I asked David when he walked into the room.

"No, not at all. This device needs to radiate directly into the skin and muscle. It's just like your annual physical—just your skivvies," he replied and adjusted the settings on the little device. I was thankful for the colorful boxers I put on that morning.

As I lay on a massage table in my studio, David moved the handheld device over my body from head to toe and read off numbers to be recorded. The device was emitting radio waves, which stimulate a self-healing process but feel like a prickling sensation.

At our next session, David used SCENAR to target areas of my body that needed treatment where Parkinson's was trying to gain a foothold. There were several spots in my body that required treatment for the healing process to begin. Towards the end of the session, the readings were higher on my upper jaw, but he could not pinpoint the problem. When I told him my dentist had just told me I needed a root canal, I realized that this SCENAR process was for real. Now I could be receptive to this new technology, and so it continued and seemed to progress more quickly.

At a subsequent session, the base of my left thumb was swollen and tender. My doctor thought it was arthritis and said that if it continued to feel sensitive, we should x-ray it and possibly see a hand specialist. When I showed David the injured thumb, he applied SCENAR to the problem area; to my surprise, after one treatment, the swelling was considerably reduced and the flexibility was noticeably improved. Who would have thought this little device would have such a dramatic effect?

HIT THE SHOWERS: RELAXATION TECHNIQUES

David and Gayla Burnett

Acupuncture

Acupuncture is a highly effective technique that generates a self-healing process in the body. Acupuncture involves the insertion of extremely thin needles through the skin at strategic points to treat pain and to balance and harmonize the body's processes. You need to identify a therapist that has the experience to understand the game plan.

Therapeutic Massage

Massage uses touch through rubbing or kneading of parts of the body to aid circulation and relax the muscles. Massage is one of the oldest, simplest forms of therapy.

The basic goal of massage therapy is to help the body heal itself and to increase health and well-being. There are many health benefits to receiving massage therapy on a regular basis. Massage helps to relieve stress, encourages relaxation, helps to manage pain, relaxes muscles, and improves flexibility.

ONE PLAY AT A TIME

The offense outlined here is the heart and soul of dealing with Parkinson's. It is lengthy and detailed with all of the treatment strategies, which can become overwhelming. Take small steps and focus on elements that will have a profound impact; that will be noticeable to not only yourself, but also to others. My journey to self-healing began with a commitment to fitness. For the first time in four years, I could actually see progress, which boosted my self-worth.

Don't try to change everything at once. Just integrate one coach or player into your game plan at a time and pay attention to the results of each adjustment. Otherwise, you will be overwhelmed and tempted to quit before you see the results.

THE OFFENSIVE TEAM IS PUSHING BACK

"Bob, I have to tell you, I'm pretty impressed by your progress. I didn't think you could do it." David's smart-aleck tone was mixed in only to soften the truth he was speaking.

"Yeah, I know. I'm surprising myself too. I can't believe how much better I feel after just a short time following the playbook you gave me."

"Well, I think it would be good for you to begin keeping a journal, my friend. You're getting enough significant results that it might help you to start setting some stronger goals, trying some new plays, and keeping track of the results you get with each one."

"Okay, you got it." I went home, eager to begin. But no one could have prepared me for benefits of this new part of my protocol.

The Game Plan was achieving unexpected results!

PAY ATTENTION TO THE SCOREBOARD

"It's not wanting to win that makes you a winner, it's refusing to fail." —PEYTON MANNING

They played hard defensively in the first quarter and even harder offensively in the second quarter, but the coach isn't about to let up on them.

"You guys are kicking butt and taking names out there. Defense looks great. Offense looks great. That play, you two," he nods in the direction of the quarterback and the running back, "what you overcame in the second quarter was damn well inspiring."

He pauses to let it all sink in before continuing, "Guys, it's time for you to pay close attention to that scoreboard and clock. Don't take your eyes off of them, even when we have the ball. Do you hear me? Pay attention to what's working on the field and between certain players, and run with it. Don't give them an inch!" he exclaims as he throws his hand out to start the huddle.

When all the players' hands are in, one on top of the other, they all shout, "One, two, three, team!"

They run back onto the field, ready to play at a whole new level.

"WOW. LOOK HOW FAR I'VE COME."

In 2011, my commitment to *The Parkinson's Playbook* was focused on the treatment strategies in the Second Quarter Offensive Game Plan. I had years of bad habits and physical limitations to overcome. It took time and dedication to make changes in my fight against Parkinson's, as it will for you.

Since work was off the table, it became easier to create a routine in the morning and stick to the sequence for the multitude of medications and supplements required. The afternoon was devoted to getting out of the house and hitting the gym to work on my fitness plan. Just getting out of the house and interacting with other people was the first step in making the transition from working at a job to a new life devoted to healing my body.

The gym is about two miles from my house and near my former downtown workplace, so initially, I dressed like I was going to work to create some semblance that life had not changed.

But let me tell you, being the new person at the gym was intimidating, as I was surrounded by a bunch of buff gym rats.

I should turn around, get the hell out of here, and go home. I was feeling totally inadequate with my baggy shorts and t-shirts, worn to hide my fat belly. *I bet they're thinking that I'm just a roly-poly guy with a long way to go ... that I'll probably give up in two weeks.*

But I didn't give up.

The yoga sessions were in a separate room; a safe place, out of sight and private. What I liked immediately about the yoga philosophy is that it is called a "practice;" there is no competition with others in the class. If I couldn't do a pose, it was okay because it was only practice. Progress is the key. I was not judged, even if it took months to master a pose.

When the gym rats saw me at the gym on a regular basis and witnessed how the exercise and yoga classes were starting to change my body shape (it took about six months), they began to comment on the progress I was making: "Have you lost weight?" Just those few words boosted my spirits.

One day, I was late for yoga class, as my neurologist appointment ran longer than expected. When class ended, I asked the yoga instructor if I could speak to the class about why I was late. The entire class waited to hear what I had to say: "The neurologist said that if he saw me on the street today, he would never know I had Parkinson's."

My yoga teacher almost cried hearing my announcement, and how I went on to explain that fitness was a significant part of turning around my health. The entire class came up to me and gave their support to keep up the fight against Parkinson's. The experience was heartwarming and gratifying!

WOW-ING THE CROWD

My wife's art opening occurred almost a full year after I committed to the Second Quarter Game Plan, and several friends that I had not seen in quite a while were shocked by how good I looked. Several of them even walked by, not recognizing me at all. When I greeted them, they would take a step back in disbelief, their eyes wide as saucers, heads shaking and voices quivering. They were truly speechless. They could not believe such a dramatic change could happen in a person fighting Parkinson's disease. The last time they saw me, I was shaking like a leaf, hunched over, and on a downward spiral. They were completely awed and elated when they realized it was me standing there, upright, slim, and steady.

That experience was a big deal for me—a defining moment, proving beyond a doubt that the hard work I was doing was making an obvious impact on my health and my outlook.

Damn, I might actually win this game.

MY PERSONAL SCOREBOARD

Remember, the whole point of this game with Parkinson's is to push back the symptoms and score easier breaths, movement, days, and wonderful moments of your life.

As I look back on the last few years, it becomes really obvious that like a good Head Coach, I paid attention to what was happening on the field and in my body. And when I noticed that one of my plays (activities or practices) was getting me further down the field than the others, I not only continued to run that play, I made note of it for future games in my journal.

One of the best things I did was begin to journal my goals and my progress—and yes, even my turn-overs, whether they were fumbles (dropping the ball) or pass interceptions (giving the ball back to the opposing team). The side benefit of journaling was going back in time and realizing the strides the Game Plan was making on my life!

Here is a bit of a highlight reel:

Wednesday 23rd

Six-month meeting with my general practitioner went well. We are reducing cholesterol and blood pressure medications by half—no problem doing it, as my recent bloodwork has shown quite an improvement. I brought a couple of emails to colleagues, and he thought I should write a book about what we were doing. He said that others are not doing the whole scope of what we have implemented. He felt it would be an inspiration to others on how we have changed my life.

The neurologist has cut Artane Parkinson's medication by one-third; he also felt good with the reduction of Cymbalta.

Slept good last night.

Happy day on Wednesday.

Thursday: No wine in the evening. Felt good the next day, slept for 9 hours straight!

GAME DAY

Tailgating

The first item on the pre-game checklist is to get your game outfit ready and load up the grill, chairs, and serving table. The most important items are the tickets, and I get my wife to double-check on those before we leave home for each game. We arrive at the parking lot outside of the stadium several hours before kickoff to enjoy the tailgate camaraderie with a group of friends who come together to get pumped up for each home game. We talk up how great our team will do and trash the opposing team. Our food and beverage menu includes burgers, brats, chips and dips, potato salad, coleslaw, beans, brownies (in Colorado, you need to ask if they are magic brownies!), cookies, and, of course, beer, margaritas, and tequila shots. It's a family affair of Broncos fanatics, a ritual, and a festive atmosphere!

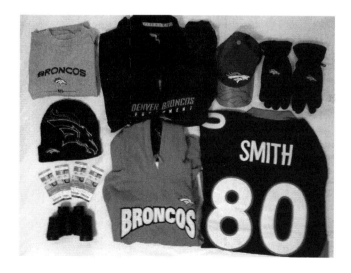

Planning ahead and staying prepared is as important for those with Parkinson's as it is for any sports fan getting ready for game day.

FOOTBALL PRE-GAME WARM-UP

Football players start the pre-game warm-up period with stretching to loosen their muscles in preparation for the start of the game. It's just like yoga class, with the captains leading the team through the warm-up routine. Recently I was surprised to find a picture in the newspaper showing football players using a down dog yoga pose as part of their pregame warm-up routine. Wow! Yoga is going mainstream!

PARKINSON'S PRE-GAME WARM-UP

Just like football players, you need to warm up your muscles prior to the exercise class to avoid pulling a muscle, which could be a setback in your fitness program. There are many types and variations for stretching prior to a workout. There are a couple of warm-up routines that consist of a short period on the stationary bike and/or treadmill, followed by several of the joint-freeing exercises (find them at Mukunda Stiles, www.yogatherapycenter.org) that seem to work for me. The stationary bike for ten to thirty minutes is a good beginning. Start out slow and gradually build up your speed, and don't be intimidated by a gym rat next to you. Hold your head high and enjoy that you are there working out.

The treadmill is the same approach as the bike. Walking on the treadmill seems too easy, but I have learned that you can hear your feet shuffling, so it makes you concentrate on lifting your feet so you stride with a good cadence. Soon you will notice a difference in how you walk in general.

FOOTBALL KICK-OFF AND FIRST DOWNS

The winner of the coin flip chooses whether they are going to kick off or receive to begin the game. The team that starts on offense gets four plays to make a first down of ten yards and another set of downs in their march to score a touchdown, which counts for seven points. The field is one hundred yards in length; and if you start on the twenty-yard line on your half of the field, your team needs to make eight first downs (ten yards) to score a touchdown. Longer plays than ten yards lessens the distance to score. The slang for a First Down is "moving the chains," as you want to keep the momentum moving forward to score a touchdown.

PARKINSON'S FIRST DOWNS

INITIAL PLAY GAINS THREE YARDS: I was having pain in the soles and toes of my feet. I tried several types of shoes that were designed to provide relief for foot pain, everything from rocker shoes to Rockport's. During a yoga class, there was one pose that was very difficult and painful from my toes to my thighs. After several sessions, I found that I was experiencing less pain in the soles and toes of my feet.

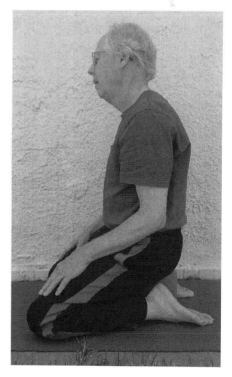

Prior to a yoga session, I often take a few minutes to gradually loosen my thigh and foot ligaments. Before I get in bed, I often apply a joint balm to relieve the tension and rub my heels to avoid deep cracks that can be painful. Now I can sit down on my heels and my feet do not hurt.

Stretching thighs and feet

SECOND PLAY GAINS FOUR YARDS: My toe next to my little toe was curling under the middle toe, which is not an easy fix. I had three visits to my general physician, without much help. But at a yoga-supply store, I found toe socks that separate your toes. It took a while to retrain my toes to be in their natural position, but it worked. The other benefit is that I am able to spread my toes so they have a gap between them, which aids in my balance.

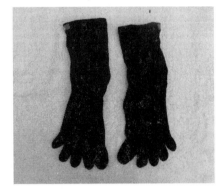

Toe socks

THIRD DOWN GAINS FOUR YARDS: Every day, you need to make small gains in your health. Little things are constantly coming up for you to deal with, as Parkinson's does not care about your well-being. I am always dealing with new issues, and what I have experienced is that little things become a big deal if you do not address them aggressively.

At a wedding in New Jersey, my wife dragged me onto the dance floor with my stylish boots, which were not made for dancing a half dozen songs. Needless to say, by the time we got back to the hotel, I could hardly walk. Since we were out of town, the next day's mission was to buy a pair of walking shoes. Since then, I have been using a roller ball to work the ligaments. My doctor pointed out that I should not walk barefoot or with just socks or slippers without an arch support. Now when I get up, the first thing I do is work on my feet and put on my casual sneaker shoe. It's made all the difference in the world. Pretty good-looking feet!

Keep making strides... it's a *first down*!!!

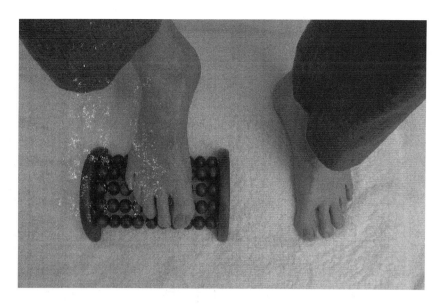

Roller ball

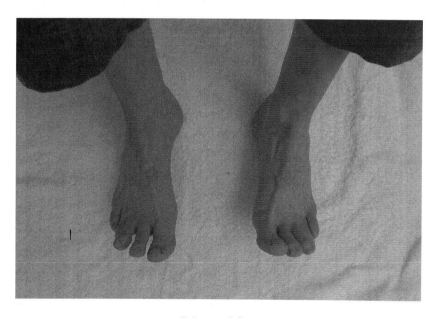

Point and flex

FOOTBALL PUNTING

When a team does not make a first down after three plays, they have the choice to "go for it" on the fourth play to reach the ten yard distance needed to receive another four plays and continue on the march to score a touchdown. If they fail to get a first down on the fourth try, the ball goes to the opposing team, and the other team gains a big advantage by having a shorter distance to score a touchdown. The alternative is to kick the ball (punt the ball) to the opposing team's half of the field, making it a longer distance for them to score a touchdown.

PARKINSON'S PUNTING

Prior to beginning the playbook strategy for Parkinson's disease, I actually stopped seeing the neurologist for a long period of time. I was tired of being nauseous and not seeing results. I did not want to believe medicine was going to make me better. What a mistake! Not taking the medications he prescribed was a setback. I gave Parkinson's the opportunity to take over the ball on my part of the field. However, after seeing the benefits of the playbook in action, leveraging fitness, muscular therapy, and mental strategies became my most effective plays.

FOOTBALL FIELD GOAL

After three plays, if the team is not able to get a first down, the offensive team can choose to kick the ball through the uprights and score three points. It's a consolation, but it gives the team the benefit of adding three points to the scoreboard.

PARKINSON'S FIELD GOAL

Equating Parkinson's to a field goal has many similarities to traditional medications and the relationship to fitness. Each year, the fitness program correlates to a decrease in your medications for cholesterol, blood pressure, and hormones, and even your Parkinson's medications. They are small steps, but they are steps that decrease wear and tear on your body. It just feels great when the doctor says we can reduce a particular medication after looking at the most recent blood work. They are incremental gains over time, but hugely encouraging milestones.

FOOTBALL FUMBLES AND INTERCEPTIONS

Turnovers give the ball back to the opponent.

There are two game-changing plays a team can make that will have a profound effect on the outcome of the game:

- Fumbles occur when a player literally drops the ball and the other team pounces on it. The fumble sets the team back—they have one less opportunity to score points, as the opposing team now has the ball.

- Interceptions are similar to a fumble, except the ball is thrown by the quarterback. The opposing team catches the ball intended for the receiver, so the ball goes to the opposing team.

Fumbles and interceptions are like accidents. You can't go back and change the outcome. The debilitating effect of an accident can have a major impact in holding the line to keep pushing back Parkinson's.

PARKINSON'S FUMBLES AND INTERCEPTIONS

Accidents create turnovers. As time goes on, the ability to do simple physical tasks is taken for granted in the early stages of Parkinson's. I say to myself, "No problem, I have done that several times." But the reality is that now my balance and coordination are off, and the other physical limitations make it very easy to stumble and hurt myself. The following photos show what happened when I was hurrying to clean up after painting a wall outside of our house. I was late, and all of a sudden, I tripped on the basement steps and landed face-down. At the time, I could not tell you where I fell, but I called my wife and told her I that I had fallen and was bleeding. I ended up in the emergency room. The next day, I needed to see the dentist because my two front teeth were loose. All of this happened two days before my nephew's wedding. *Way to go, Bob!* I looked like a wreck. What a way to meet the new relatives.

The frustrating part is, I knew better. A year earlier, we were having old friends from out of town over for dinner, and I was the designated grill master. Earlier in the day, I installed spotlights for the grill area; and when I looked up, I saw that I had one more screw to put in. I hopped up on our firewood container, three to four-feet high. I knew as soon as I got up on the table that I was off-balance and headed down. I knocked over a large potted plant container. The pot hit the stairs first, and I was second. I landed face down in the dirt, which helped to cushion the fall. I was lucky that I did not break any bones, but I did end up with a lump the size of an egg on the side of my head, which went away in a few hours. My neurologist, needless to say, was not pleased.

There are times when I see a bruise on my shoulder or leg and cannot remember how it happened. When I do it a second time, "Oh, it was the side of the door or the open dishwasher door." The point is that you have to be alert, even when just walking around the house. It can happen simply walking down the stairs and thinking wrongly that you are at the bottom. You lurch forward and are relieved that you did

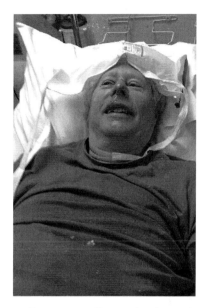 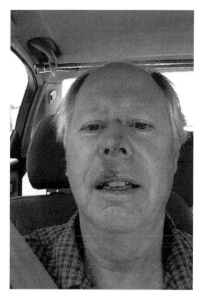

Emergency Room check-up   The aftermath

not take a tumble. The fitness work does pay off with better balance and coordination, but you still have to be careful.

What I have learned from accidents is that you can seriously hurt yourself, and recovering might take a while. The lack of movement gives Parkinson's the opportunity to increase its grip, making it harder to recover. It is imperative that you are careful and do not take unnecessary risks. Your caregivers also need to recognize that you cannot do the same things now and should be aware of possible injury situations.

FOOTBALL TOUCHDOWNS

The team's objective is to score more touchdowns and field goals (to score points) than the opposing team in order to win the game. A touchdown is when a team moves the ball down the field with continuous first downs and crosses the goal line. It is not easy to go the length of the field with the defense bent on stopping them from getting first downs. Touchdowns are not easy to make, and it is gratifying and thrilling when they finally cross that line.

PARKINSON'S TOUCHDOWNS

My son-in-law runs a river rafting operation on the Colorado River Center in Colorado, which has given me the opportunity to be an active participant. On some days, I just paddle and enjoy the scenery. On days when the water level is down, I have had the chance to take over the guide's duty of rowing and steering the raft, and impressed the guide with my strength to handle the raft without difficulty. Fitness helps you in many ways as you remain active with biking, skiing, running, or just good old walking. Strive to score touchdowns—it's how you win against Parkinson's. *Yes, we scored!*

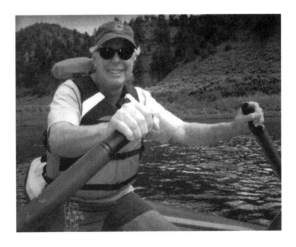

Rafting the Colorado River

AWAY GAMES: TRAVEL

Often, just the thought of traveling becomes a greater hurdle than it needs to be. The key to traveling with Parkinson's is pre-planning and anticipating the unexpected.

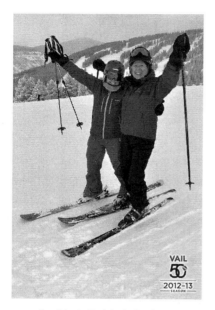
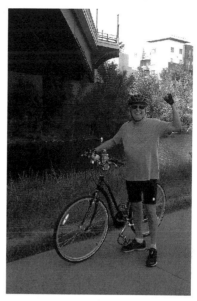

In 2013, I skied the best
in my life!

Easy on and off bike frame

Pre-planning cannot be overlooked. It is the first priority. Once, when I was leaving for a trip, the stress and anxiety were so overwhelming that nausea hit and I headed to the bathroom minutes before heading to the airport. Everyone was on me, saying, "Let's go! We are going to miss the plane!" And that *has* happened . . . not a pleasant way to start your vacation.

The first step is to organize your medications and supplements to see if there are sufficient pills for the trip. Your pharmacy can order a vacation supply for the duration of your trip, but make sure you start this process two weeks in advance, as it is inevitable that your doctor will need to renew your scripts. Refer back to your renewal chart we discussed earlier to help with what you will need. There are great travel containers that can help you manage your pills and supplements while on the road.

Whether flying or driving, I do not book a flight or leave home before 11:00 am, and I arrive no later than 6:00 pm. Those early morning flights just create a lot of stress and anxiety, and I say it's better to enjoy your trip from the beginning.

I take a backpack or small suitcase with all my medications, snacks, power bars, whole meal packets, and water. Don't check them, as they could end up getting lost, and then you would be in big trouble. Airlines do not have a problem with your rolling pharmacy, but it's good to be prepared. You can have your doctor write a letter regarding your condition and a list of medications in case you get stopped at security, and it's a good idea to have all of your doctors' phone numbers handy.

Another tidbit is to take those little baggies for a whole day's regimen of pills and put them in your pocket for easy access. You don't want to be caught stranded on the runway for hours and have withdrawals. I do the same thing for being out and about on a daily basis. It's a priority the first thing in the morning to get those little pill packets ready.

You should not leave home without your yoga mat and band. Even

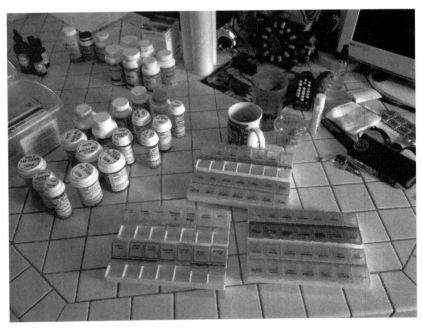

Pill management and pill containers

on the road, taking a few minutes for an exercise program is important to maintain your fitness level. Walking will be a part of sightseeing and visiting new places and can serve as your cardio exercise. I make a copy of the exercise programs to serve as a reminder to stay on track every day. Doing a little bit of your program will offset sitting all day in a plane, car, or RV.

When booking lodging, we try to stay at places that serve a mini-breakfast—enough so that you have food in your stomach for your pills to land before you get ready for the day's adventure. It helps prevent unnecessary searches for restaurants and keeps you on schedule. Another option is to book an apartment where you can live like you are at home. B&B's are another neat option for a "home away from home" setting.

Two weeks prior to the trip, organize your clothes in a spare room; the night before the trip, lay out what you are going to wear to start the trip. Pre-planning prevents being up until midnight with last-minute struggles. Get a good night's sleep! In the morning, all you have to do is shower, put on your clothes, and walk out the door with your suitcase. There's no stress or anxiety, and you are ready to enjoy the trip!

SCOREBOARD BY YEAR

At the beginning of my game with Parkinson's, I was at the bottom of the pile, both physically and mentally. There was nowhere to go but up with only a ray of hope. Parkinson's was winning the battle in the league standings, and we were looking at another losing season.

The scoreboard for Parkinson's is expressed as a wheel divided into slices of my daily life (shown as percentages). At the beginning of the game, I felt like much of my life was out of my control. Traditional medicine was barely able to keep me afloat, and exercise was a negligible part of the fight against Parkinson's. As you'll see, over time, the Scoreboard started to change, until one day, my prior life was barely recognizable.

2011 SCOREBOARD

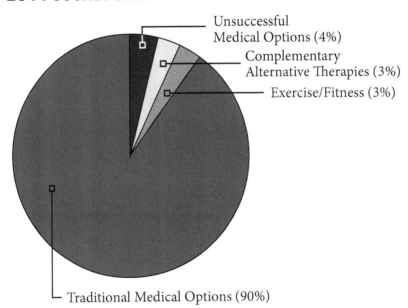

Unsuccessful
Medical Options (4%)

Complementary
Alternative Therapies (3%)

Exercise/Fitness (3%)

Traditional Medical Options (90%)

When the scoreboard looked like this, I was out of control with worsening symptoms (including tremors, depression, behavior issues, speech impediment, gait problems, lack of stamina, and fear).

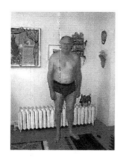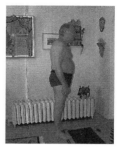

Physical condition in February 2011; starting weight: 182 pounds

2011 Goals

Playbook Strategy: 60% Traditional Medicine and 40% Complementary and Alternative Medicine (fitness, nutrition, supplements and alternative therapies)

- Improve overall health
- Dedicate four to five days each week to yoga and cardiovascular exercise
- Overcome stress and anxiety
- Reduce right-side tremors

February 17, 2011 was my last day of employment and the beginning of my three years on disability. During the first two weeks, it seemed like I spent the whole time sleeping. I was fortunate that my company had the foresight to have a disability policy for the business partners, in addition to a companywide policy to cover my salary. The coverage provided the opportunity to completely step away from work and totally immerse myself in the goal of getting my life on the right track without the stress and anxiety of the workplace or serious money concerns. Part of the requirement to receive disability compensation was that I could not have any work-related contact with my former employer.

Also in February, I started the Game Plan philosophy developed by the Burnetts, which (as you've seen) included Bowen Therapy and a supplement/nutrition plan to augment the traditional Parkinson's medications. My physical fitness level had been progressively deteriorating each year, even with Parkinson's treatment, and my new fitness program focused on alleviating Parkinson's physical limitations, including weight gain, rounded posture, shuffling feet, and the loss of balance, coordination, and stamina.

Initially, I started the exercise program with the Joint Freeing Series (found at www.yogatherapycenter.org) three days a week to increase flexibility, and gradually I transitioned to a yoga practice three days a week, a personal trainer the fourth day, and the fifth day devoted to cardio and strength-building work. As my body was responding, it was clear that my dedication and commitment to the Game Plan was becoming visible at a steady rate. I probably have said it many times, but this could not have happened without my wife and a team of experts who were so supportive, especially during the early stages of retooling my health. The creative approach of the Game Plan gave me a path that I could follow to improve my life.

It took a year to achieve my short-term goals, and that did not fully happen until I stopped working and could devote the energy necessary to make a difference in slowing down the Parkinson's progression. I have achieved a good handle on the physical part, but the mental part still has room for improvement. As you can see, the wellness program has taken as much work as the passion you typically put into your profession. The motto now is, "Leave no stone unturned in the pursuit of a better quality of life." My daughter lives in Vail, and the last few years I was not able to ski. My yoga therapist has helped to improve my balance, which has been a big step in helping me to tackle the slopes again.

2011 Results

General health and fitness were on an upswing and showing results both outwardly and internally.

2012 SCOREBOARD

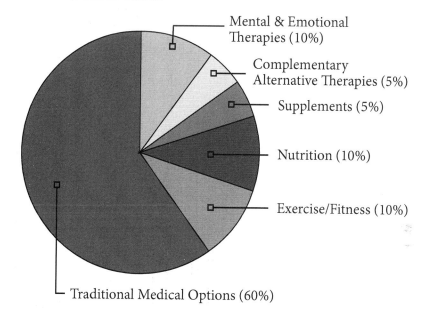

Mental & Emotional Therapies (10%)

Complementary Alternative Therapies (5%)

Supplements (5%)

Nutrition (10%)

Exercise/Fitness (10%)

Traditional Medical Options (60%)

2012 Goals

Playbook Strategy: 60% Traditional Medicine and 40% Complementary and Alternative Medicine (fitness, nutrition, supplements and alternative therapies)

- Improve overall health
- Longer waking days
- Reach out to others
- Reduce medications
- Record yoga sessions

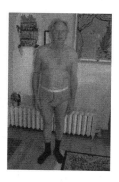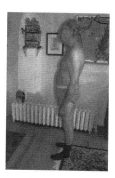

Physical condition in 2012; starting weight: 162 pounds, end of year weight: 152 pounds

This was a year of growth and accomplishments. It was a significant milestone to understand the commitment it takes to slow down Parkinson's and be at a stable position over a long period. It has taken the help of everyone on my team making contributions to help abate the downward spiral of this chronic, degenerative disease.

A turning point was experiencing full days without the negative impacts of Parkinson's. That was a wonderful feeling! I still had a tough period in the mornings, but they were becoming less and less frequent. Five days a week of fitness, targeting poses, and exercises made a difference in my balance and coordination. Our approach to exercise routines has changed from just a yoga class to a plan that also includes flexibility, stretching, cardio, and overall strength building.

2012 Results

At the start of 2012, I began with a split of 40% Complementary and Alternative Medicine and 60% going towards Traditional Medicine.

The plan had been so successful in mitigating my symptoms that at the end of 2012, I achieved a split of 60% Complementary and Alternative Medicine (the offense) and 40% Traditional Medicine (the defense).

The playbook was achieving unexpected results and my health and fitness continued to improve to the point where the physical turnaround is striking.

2013 SCOREBOARD

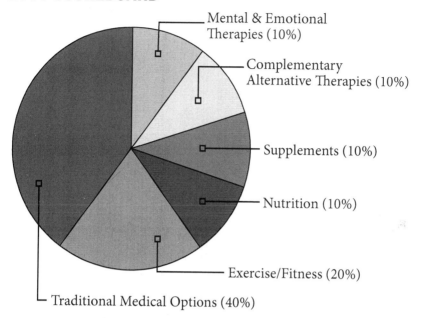

Mental & Emotional Therapies (10%)

Complementary Alternative Therapies (10%)

Supplements (10%)

Nutrition (10%)

Exercise/Fitness (20%)

Traditional Medical Options (40%)

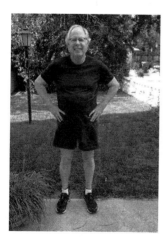
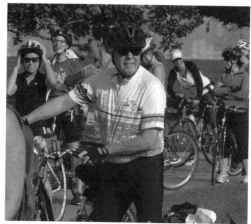

Photograph by Grace Combs Photography

Physical condition in 2013; starting weight: 152 pounds,
end of year weight: 146 pounds.

2013 Goals

Playbook Strategy: 40% Traditional Medicine and 60% Complementary and Alternative Medicine (fitness, nutrition, supplements and alternative therapies)

- Continue to improve overall health

- Initiate and develop a happiness pattern

My yoga therapist, Alana, mentioned I should listen to a piece on happiness from the TED Talks video series (www.ted.com) by Shawn Anchor called "The Happy Secret to Better Work". Since first viewing the video, I have probably watched it five times. It spoke to me as a clear path in dealing with Parkinson's. It encompasses most of the traits I am following now and emphasized that the key to a brighter future, even during the tough days, is to bring fun, happiness, and mastery into my life while helping others realize they can also make changes in their lives. The video suggests it will take the brain three weeks to rewire the pathways to happiness, which is not a long time if you are diligent and focused on improving your quality of life!

Here's what I decided to add to my offense game:

- Journaling: Review what I'm grateful for every day

- Meditation

- Random acts of kindness

- Listening to music

Looking back, Febuary 2011 was when I started to accept the fact that I had Parkinson's and needed to focus my energy on dealing with a difficult disease. As each team member advised me, the cumulative input was changing my body and mind, slowly providing results. Looking at three consecutive years of photographs gave me the encouragement to move forward in my life. Things feed on one another, whether they are positive or negative. Being the "fun Bob" needed to be on my mind every hour of the day.

As I meet people who had not seen me in a while, they were astounded at how good I looked and what I was doing to make life changes. Some of their friends have Parkinson's, and they are also searching for remedies to this crippling disease. My belief is that it takes a diversified team of professionals working in concert to slow down Parkinson's. It can be done by being proactive, focused, and having the will to commit to the work, day in and day out.

2013 Results

At the start of 2013, I began with a split of 60% Complementary and Alternative Medicine and 40% going towards Traditional Medicine.

By the end of 2013, the plan exceeded my goal for the year, reaching a split of 89% going towards Complementary and Alternative Medicine (the offense) and 11% going towards Traditional Medicine (the defense).

The changes I experienced in my health and fitness for the year were beyond my expectations. I was fit, trim, lean, and flexible—right where I wanted to be. My body fat percentage was 14.5%, which is in the ideal range for my height and age!

2014 SCOREBOARD

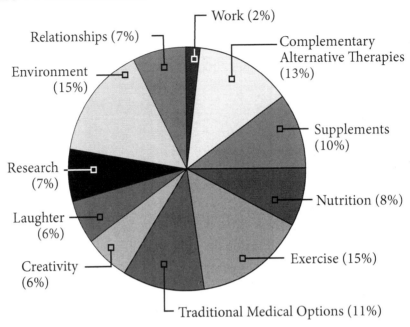

Work (2%)

Relationships (7%)

Complementary Alternative Therapies (13%)

Environment (15%)

Supplements (10%)

Research (7%)

Nutrition (8%)

Laughter (6%)

Creativity (6%)

Exercise (15%)

Traditional Medical Options (11%)

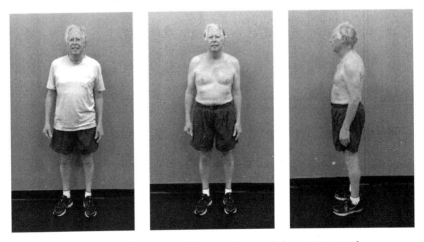

Physical condition in 2014; starting weight: 146 pounds, end of year weight: 142 pounds.

2014 Goals

- Fine-tune my fitness program
- Use video and photography to help evaluate my progress so that I can see it visually
- Increase my happiness
- Improve overall health (weight goal: 140 to 150 pounds)

The 2014 (and beyond) goal is to create a consistent pattern that still emphasizes a fitness program of yoga and exercise, mental health (mastery and pleasure), attention to medications and what they are or are not doing, and enjoying time with family. Dealing with depression, anxiety, and stress continue to be an ongoing issue. Meeting with my psychologist helped to relieve and lessen the mental part of Parkinson's. Music also started to play a role in providing a way to focus my thoughts on something soothing and relaxing.

This year's achievements included several successes from skiing (which is unheard of for a person with Parkinson's), the 30.1-mile charity fundraiser Pedaling 4 Parkinson's, and guiding a raft—all of which are on the physical part of managing Parkinson's.

2014 Results

I continued a split of 89% Complementary and Alternative Medicine (the offense) and 11% going towards Traditional Medicine (the defense). I was able to maintain this balance for the full calendar year. In looking ahead to future goals, I have found that maintaining the current level of fitness will be the challenge; once I got there, I could tell I was backsliding. Recommitment is now a daily reality.

FOUR-YEAR LOOK BACK

Looking back at my progress since 2011 is gratifying and rewarding. I find it uplifting!

Reviewing the photographs as I worked on this book, I noticed that my feet look like I still walk like a duck. This is another challenge to deal with, and it highlights the benefit of recording your body's evolution.

After years of weight loss, I was swimming in my clothes. Be prepared to update your wardrobe. Except for the cost of new outfits, you will look and feel good about your new body.

AREAS OF IMPROVEMENT: THE CROWD CHEERS

From Alana Foeller, Yoga Therapist, Ayurveda Practitioner, Registered Nurse

Bob's wellness program stays strong!

BALANCE: Improvement with lunge poses and single-leg standing poses

SHOULDER/CHEST: More open, with greater shoulder range of motion (ROM)

UPPER BACK: Less rounding in the thoracic spine

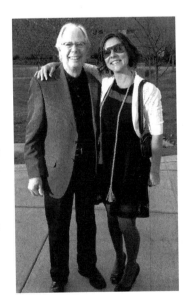

DEEPER BREATHING

- Much more movement in chest and belly on inhalation
- Able to relax on exhalation
- Breath is more fluid; not gasping for air like before

ANKLE AND KNEE JOINTS

- Range of motion better
- Noticeable flexibility improvement in ankles and feet
- Can sit back on heels without a block!

FEET: Able to separate (spread) toes

SLEEPING: 7–8 hours a day

From Dr. Stanley Kerstein, MD

In thirty years of practice, I have seen only a handful of people who have been able to deal with Parkinson's, and Bob is one.

From David Burnett, Bowen Practitioner

On a visit to Bob's house, I noticed he was sitting on a bar stool at the kitchen table. One leg was on the footrest and the other leg was resting on the next chair, so that his spine was twisted and his head was forward. I suggested Bob use a step stool to rest his feet at a good height, which allowed him to get closer to the table, keeping his feet aligned and making him sit up straighter in a better posture. The last tidbit was to put a phone book under his laptop to help keep his head back. On a subsequent visit, I noticed his improvement and remarked, "Damn! He actually did it!"

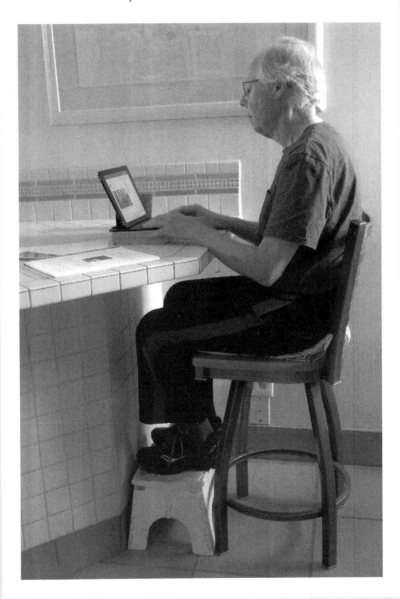

NOVEMBER 2015: It is very difficult to know when to stop writing and move on to the publishing phase. I feel the next paragraph will be the conclusion. There are a few thoughts regarding where I am at this point in dealing with Parkinson's:

- There are times that I am not aware that I have Parkinson's.

- I am sleeping seven to eight hours a night, with only one bathroom trip.

- Happiness is gradually being incorporated daily.

- My medications are at a stable point.

- It has been several months since I felt nausea in the morning after taking my pills and supplements.

- My quality of life is on an upswing.

- Lately, I have been experiencing dry mouth. I started using an oral rinse to help with the condition. What I found was that it was a result of dehydration, and drinking water has helped to mitigate the condition.

- Anxiety and stress still occur, but for a shorter time period, as meditation and breathing exercises help. The mental part is the hardest to deal with, and should be right up there with fitness as part of dealing with Parkinson's daily.

- Fitness sessions five days a week keep me flexible.

- Don't assume that the Playbook is easy. It's not. It takes a lot of consistent and committed effort.

- Family support and caring for each other has been what makes it all worthwhile.

- As Bob Marley used to say, "Be happy."

- On days when I don't have an exercise session because I feel physically or emotionally imbalanced, or when I am traveling, I work on seated poses only (no standing poses) and concentrate on relaxation with long *savasana* (relaxing pose) and deep breathing. I emphasize the deep breathing, using a beaded necklace and moving one bead for each breath.

- Generally, the past year or so, I have only gotten up once or not at all in my sleep pattern. When I have too many cocktails, I am up three or four times. I have noticed that sound sleep begins between 2 am and 3 am.

MORE TO THE SCOREBOARD

Even with all the progress and the crowd cheering, it's still a lot of work to keep the physical and mental health steady, and David was paying careful attention to this area as my coach and my friend.

"Well, I'm glad you're feeling better physically. It looks like that's helping to offset the depression." It was a question wrapped in observation.

"Yes, it is. Quite a bit. But some days, I still . . ." My voice trailed off as I felt traces of depression and rage simultaneously make themselves known in my throat.

"What are you doing to manage the mental and emotional, Bob?"

"I don't know. Do you have suggestions?"

"Well, yes, I do."

And so, we began to discuss the need for your MVP to enter the game.

FOURTH QUARTER

PLAY YOUR SECRET WEAPONS (MVPs)

"Always have four things in life:

Something to do.

Someone to love.

Something to hope for.

Something to believe in." —LOU HOLTZ

The players huddle together before the last quarter.

"Alright, guys, the third quarter was great. You're all looking good out there and playing as a team. Now it's time to bring out our secret weapons." He takes a breath before revealing the players he is going to put in and the plays he's been working on, but they all know who the secret weapons are.

They are the Most Valuable Players (the MVPs) because they have the clearest minds and nerves of steel. No matter what kind of pressure the rest of the team is feeling, these guys are always clear-headed and calm. They operate "in the zone" every time they are on the field. And the coach always brings them in at the right time and gives them the perfect plays to finish off the game.

He makes eye contact with the two MVPs he decides to send onto the field and says, "Okay, you two. I want you to . . ."

The whole team nods, pumped with excitement about this last quarter. They can taste victory!

A NEW COACH

"Welcome to my office, Bob. Please make yourself comfortable," he invited as he extended his hand in the direction of the client chair. I was immediately grateful for two things: one, he was wearing khakis and a nice button-up shirt, and second, he was not asking me to lie down on a couch. (Oh, the ideas the movies put in our heads!)

Once I was seated comfortably, he continued. "I'd like to start this get-to-know-each-other session by sharing a little bit about myself, my specialties, and how we could work together."

Whew. I'm so glad I don't have to do all the talking. I relaxed a little into my seat and listened attentively, trying to ignore the anxiety that was tightening my chest and creeping up my shoulders.

He went on to share about his many degrees and specialties as a psychologist, one of which was successfully working with people with behavioral issues, as well as people dealing with cognitive and affective challenges—or, in simple terms, behavioral addictions. When he mentioned those words, I felt my stomach tighten and my legs go a little numb. I knew this feeling—it was the same feeling I had whenever I felt I was about to be "found out." It was *shame.*

He must have noticed that I sat forward in my chair, as he spent quite a bit of time sharing about the work with those engaged in unhealthy and self-destructive behaviors, noting intentionally that he had never worked with a Parkinson's patient before.

I felt relief wash over me from head to toe. *He's going to be able to help me with these compulsive and mood-altering behaviors (brought on by my Parkinson's medications) that have wreaked havoc in my marriage, my finances, and my life.*

"So, that's a little about me," he smiled and nodded toward me, pausing before, "How about you, Bob? I'd love it if you would share a little about yourself, your life before Parkinson's and since, and where you would like to start with our work together."

His calm presence, kindness, and curiosity made me feel so safe that I quickly found myself sharing feelings and behavior problems that I never imagined I would share with anyone. I talked about the anxiety, depression, stress, and compulsive behavior, and its medication protocol. As I spoke, I felt both fearful and relieved to finally get all this crap off my chest to someone who wasn't going to be hurt or angry in response. But most importantly, I felt heard—*known*—for the first time in a long time. He wasn't jotting notes. He was looking me in the eyes, and I couldn't see anything but sympathy and kindness.

When the session ended and I'd wiped the tears from my eyes, shaken his hand gratefully, and walked back to my car, I realized that there wouldn't be a fast and easy fix; but with time, there could be a lot of relief and progress.

THE MENTAL AND EMOTIONAL GAME

One of the harder aspects of Parkinson's is depression. It does not have a specific time of the day or night that it visits, but it is set in motion when anxiety and stress are present. People with Parkinson's need to produce dopamine, a neurotransmitter that is largely responsible for proper movement, neurological function, and, you guessed it, feelings of happiness. The medications they offer work to trick the brain into producing dopamine, or making it believe that it has enough. Yet, as I've shared, getting the medications right is tricky.

Without the dopamine, anxiety and depression creep in and take hold as one loses control over their physical movement, their emotions, and their life.

It doesn't help that we are barraged with all the bad things on TV and in newspapers and magazines. Negative stuff is all around us and our brain is overloaded with it, whether we have Parkinson's or not. But those of us with Parkinson's need an even stronger daily, and sometimes hourly, input of inspiration to repeat the feelings of hope over and over to fuel happiness instead of negativity, despair, and anxiety. The TED Talk video mentioned in the Third Quarter ("The Happy Secret to Better Work" by Shawn Anchor) pointed out that through positive psychology, we can retrain our brain to focus on the good and fun stuff.

MOST VALUABLE PLAYER (MVP)

As I worked with the psychologist over the course of several sessions, we developed tools that were quite different than the fitness routines I was developing. These were positive psychological tools that helped me to develop happiness and self-efficacy and win the game against depression and anxiety. These tools helped me to increase my dopamine level and decrease my depression—results that my regular medications could not achieve for me.

During difficult times, when the stakes are high and the opposition is intense, the MVPs on your team come forward to help you deal with the mental and emotional game. They are the specialists in their field who can guide you in the transition from a lost identity to a new path.

As I worked with my MVP Coach, the psychologist, I started to identify and develop the Most Valuable Players on my team—tools, skills, and practices that I could throw on the field when the going was getting tough and Parkinson's was pushing back with anxiety and depression. The two significant plays created by the MVPs were what the Psychologist called "mastery" and "pleasure."

MASTERY

The way I see it, the goal of mastery is two-fold. The first part is becoming the master of the parts of your life where control has been lost: movement, feelings, and behaviors. We worked to develop tools and skills such as the pocket cards and breathing (more on this below) that would help me become the master of areas where I had begun to feel powerless.

The second part of mastery is keeping your brain moving and grooving with goals and actions to achieve them. I had a very successful career as a landscape architect, building a successful business and creating beautiful environments for forty years; and then, almost overnight, the opportunity for goal achievement and accomplishment (outside of just trying to feel better) disappeared. They say that "without vision, people perish," and I found it to be true for me emotionally. I really missed the excitement of coming up with what appeared to be unachievable goals and then developing solutions to materialize the vision. Setting new goals to master keeps my brain working and focused on things in my life other than Parkinson's.

Mastery: Pocket Cards

To help with the compulsive behaviors that had been brought on by the Parkinson's medications, we listed all the bad side effects they created on a pocket-sized card. On the reverse side, we listed the consequences of my actions. I kept the card in my pocket so that whenever bad thoughts or impulses came into my head, I could pull out the card. It would serve as a reminder of what would happen if I continued on that path. As time progressed, these simple note cards were a support device when nobody was around to say, "Bob, what are you doing?"

Mastery: Breathing

We also started to practice simple breathing exercises to settle my mind and create a relaxed atmosphere. I would sit with my eyes closed and, starting in my upper body, I would tense the muscles, squeezing hard then releasing. I worked from head to toe, letting go of my stress and anxiety.

To my surprise, the yoga portion of my fitness plan was using the same breathing and exercise techniques the psychologist was incorporating into our sessions. The combination of fitness, psychology, medication, supplements, muscular therapy, and improved family relations was allowing me to make great strides in living with Parkinson's.

Mastery: Laughter and a Positive Attitude

One night, we were watching "Downton Abbey" on PBS. There were several funny scenes, and my wife was laughing like crazy. At one point, she turned to me and said, "You really need to outwardly show your emotions—laugh a little, live a little, just have fun."

I realized that for some of us, it is easy to just absorb the emotion and hold it in; it takes a concerted effort to express ourselves and let it out, especially when your center for movement and happiness is as troubled as it is with us Parkinson's folks. I consciously need to remind myself: "You were a funny and fun guy—get back to that place."

As I started to pay attention to expressing myself through laughter and a positive attitude, happiness started to take over the "woe is me" feeling.

Mastery: Journaling

I've shared the importance of keeping a journal multiple times in this book, but I've always done it with the focus on tracking my progress. Well, there's another very important reason to journal: It helps you stay sane! It's a safe place to write down all of your feelings, goals, fears, and successes. I've known people to keep their journal electronically, but I've also heard plenty of people say that the process of handwriting is more helpful in processing the emotions and anchoring the effort in the brain. Obviously, handwriting can be quite a task for us Parkinson's people, so I imagine that doing what feels best to you is the appropriate system.

PLEASURE

There were so many activities that I enjoyed before Parkinson's, but now that my life was focused on surviving and pushing back this horrible disease, I stopped doing a lot of those things that brought me pleasure... and doing them just for pleasure's sake.

The truth is that so much of what you'll have to do on the field is *work*. You'll need to spend quite a bit of your time training, exercising, going to appointments, and doing all of the things I've shared in this book. But you must make time and space for pleasure and activities that make you happy. These can be solo activities, group activities, or both. Whatever lights you up—that's where to start!

Pleasure: Building a New Community

After stopping work, I had an internal identity crisis, which was triggered by someone asking, "Are you retired? How do you like retirement?" *I did not choose to be retired. Parkinson's chose it for me.* It was another downer moment. I got tired of the word "retired;" to me, it meant my past life had ended. I was at the peak of my profession, and now I was suddenly retired. *How am I to get past this point in my life? It is not fair.*

The emotion of losing your identity is staggering to your being. You need a new direction that preserves your dignity and self-worth. Many of my friends could not wait to leave the workplace for whatever reason—they hated their job, disliked their employer, couldn't handle being told what to do by a younger boss, or whatever—but it was *their choice* to leave. And they had great things ahead—plans to take their RV around the country or just lounge around without a time commitment. All of this was on *their* terms. But a Parkinson's person has many of those options and choices taken away from them before they can grasp what's happening.

Building a new community can seem like a daunting task after spending four decades of building relationships and support that are no longer a part of your world. I stumbled for several years, not having a direction in my life. The fitness program filled the void for several years, but there was still the drive to recreate the appreciation experienced from being part of a team that held aspirations and accomplishments.

I started to ask myself questions. *Work ended. Now what? Since I am not retired, how do I search for a new career? What have I always wanted to do that can still give me that same satisfaction? Can I reinvent myself to do something that is meaningful and that can have a greater purpose?* I needed to find a direction that would fit with the skills that could work around my Parkinson's restrictions. There were a couple of outlets to look at that could dovetail and not conflict with the number one priority in my life: healing myself.

The first step was connecting with the Parkinson's community. I initially found it a depressing experience. I felt like an outsider in a room of people trying to deal with Parkinson's disease with its many stages of progression. I was not ready to engage in this new community while still having feelings of denial. It was just too depressing. I needed time to address my health before I could engage others. As time passed, I was in a better place to join local and national Parkinson's organizations to offer support and lessons learned from the Playbook.

Pleasure: Past Community Outreach

The first thought was to look at past volunteer efforts during my working career for ideas. There was great satisfaction in helping others, which reinforced my sense of worth. I was involved in a multitude of organizations that provided benefits to the community, while also making new personal friendships. The community activities ranged from raising over several hundred thousand dollars in materials and labor towards the construction of the Columbine Memorial in

Colorado, to assisting in a community planting for restoring the landscape of the South Platte River Corridor in Denver, to fundraising for scholarships to students of Landscape Architecture and grants for Colorado landscape research projects.

Pleasure: Community Service Volunteer

Another community outlet might be to volunteer your time to a nonprofit group. There are a multitude of options out there. It could be a program such as Meals on Wheels for the sick or elderly, working at your local botanical garden, being an usher, helping a church group, or acting as a senior center assistant. The avenues are endless. Another approach could be coaching for youth sports, as it would be rewarding to see kids grow and enjoy being part of a team. Think of it as a way to give something back to the community, while the volunteer support can mesh with your medical condition.

Pleasure: Community

An unexpected new community opportunity occurred when my wife came across an article in the paper about an upcoming event to raise money for Parkinson's research, founded by three ladies dealing with their spouses' health issues. The event was called Pedaling4Parkinson's. My wife felt this could be a way to become active in the Parkinson's community. The money raised through this one-day bicycle ride encouraged those with Parkinson's to participate, even if they could not ride.

The whole atmosphere was positive and encouraging. I had never felt that emotional lift with my local Parkinson's organization. Maybe it was my attitude at that time, or my expectations. This was different. It made me feel like I was part of a family.

In our first year participating in the event, we jumped in feet-first. The idea was to form a team of riders, with each member tasked with raising $150 each from their friends. Needless to say, the Bob

Team came on like gangbusters; it was a task I was experienced with because of my work with other nonprofit organizations. We were an eye-popping team, finishing second in total team fundraising, and my daughter, the Team Captain, was first in individual soliciting money for the event. The support from family and friends meant a lot to me. The Bob Team was the largest group for the entire event, and it was quite a meaningful accomplishment to have everyone come together to support this worthwhile cause.

The next year, when I went to the packet pickup location, a wonderful thing happened. When I said, "I am Bob from the Bob Team," the sponsors and staff rushed forward to meet me. It was a moment of satisfaction and appreciation for being a leader in raising money for research by the Michael J. Fox Foundation. It felt good to be part of a worthwhile medical research campaign.

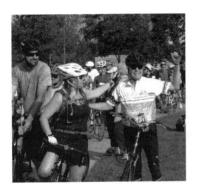 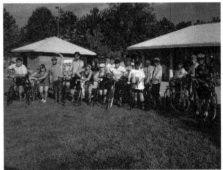

Pedaling 4 Parkinson's Fundraising Event

Pleasure: TED Videos

I highly recommend devoting some time each day or week to listening to some of the amazing people in the TED Talk videos (www.ted.com) as they share their profound stories, insights, and expertise. It truly is amazing and inspiring.

Pleasure: Music

There's always good music in the stadium before a game and during the halftime show, right? Well, I found music to be incredibly helpful in increasing my pleasure and enjoyment of life. I have different music playlists for different moods. For instance, when I am driving to yoga class, the Rolling Stones are a favorite to get me jazzed up. Another favorite is The Traveling Wilburys when I am just out and about, as the band is made up of all my favorite musicians.

For tasks that require intense concentration, such as writing, I have found it difficult to have even soft music in the background, as my brain has a hard time focusing on the task at hand. In the evening or during dinner, we often listen to Brazilian or Cuban music for its native roots and sound. All of this music improves my mood, helping me to ramp up my energy or relax it, depending on the experience I have in front of me.

Pleasure: Family and Friends

The family circle and friendship are intertwined; there is not one without the other, and the words are interchangeable. Your family is your rock. Their understanding of what you are going through makes it easier to cope with Parkinson's on a daily basis. You spend a lot of time alone, which makes having a dialogue enjoyable, even if it's just daily conversation about what happened that day.

Maintaining friendships can be a boost to your emotional well-being. After leaving the workplace, it is easy to let those ties drift away. Reconnect with those who have slipped out of your life. Make an effort to call and suggest doing something interesting or fun with them. Just meeting for lunch can be a lift that lets you into someone else's life. It's a way to have a dialogue with a friend outside of your household.

Transitioning your friendship group can take time. Think about who is in your world now and how to bring them closer. The more people you're connected with, the more expanded your support group becomes. Having a "woe is me" attitude will make it more difficult to maintain friendships. Downplay how much you talk about Parkinson's; change the subject, be upbeat in your conversations, and have an ear for others. Social media can also be a neat way to keep in touch. Facebook provides the benefit of staying abreast of what is happening with friends but also their passions and opinions. Keeping those old friends is important, and it's also important to strive to make new friendships.

I have a friend who once said, "Keep your chin up; everyone loves you." That was nice to hear.

Pleasure: A New Adventure

An idea came to mind. *Maybe there is a way to connect my interest in wine and its culture.* On many of our travels, we would often stop at vineyards for a tour and a tasting. Soon, we started to attend local tastings through our local wine and liquor store. The tastings were hosted by vineyard representatives for particular areas of the U.S., Europe, and South America. Reading about how wine is planted, harvested, bottled, and aged became a great hobby of mine. After months of reading and researching how to store wine, my first opportunity to design and build a wine cellar became a reality. The finished cellar became a new source of pride. Since then, I formed a business devoted to the design of wine cellars. The good part is that I am able to transfer what I learned in my previous work as a landscape architect to this new adventure, and gradual marketing of this new venture is underway. Locally, the reputation as "The Wine Guy" has started to take hold. Even if this new career track is low-key, it is something to hang my hat on as a worthwhile opportunity. It brings me satisfaction to chart a new path and take my mind off of Parkinson's.

Pleasure: A New Career

After years of journaling, a friend and my doctor both suggested that others might be interested in my Parkinson's journey and all of the treatment strategies that were working for me. They thought my story could be a source of hope to many. Suddenly, I was on the "author" path without fully understanding what that meant. Writing a manuscript to help others became a source of therapy and an outlet.

After several years of documenting my progress, it became evident that I was onto something besides filling a journal. Then it hit me. I was becoming an *author*. I had never been a writer, but I surprised myself with what was hidden inside my head that just needed to come out. My new occupation can fit within my day without the pressure of work deadlines and health restrictions. This truly gave me a source of pride and accomplishment. A friend said, after reviewing my manuscript, "You have reinvented yourself. You're an author!" And I realized it was time to get this out into the world.

Pleasure: Finding Happiness Everywhere

As I have been racking my brain to acknowledge everyone, from special players to special therapies, it dawned on me that they are around us every day. They do not always have titles or provide unique therapies. It is during interaction in daily living that you find them. Recently, I had cataract surgery, and for a week after having the lens in my eye replaced, I could not bend over, go to the gym, or lift anything over 25 pounds. And with only one good eye, driving was basically out of the question. It literally put my exercise program on hold. The only thing I could do to get out of the house was to go for a walk. It was winter, so I bundled up and headed out.

Two things happened, and they were different each day. Walking along the parkway, I met fellow walkers, joggers, dog walkers, and the like. I said, "Hello!" raised my hand, or occasionally met a neighbor.

It felt good, even though it was only a flicker of time. I started to make up stories about each one that passed by... where they were going, whether I would see them on the return route, and if I would see them the next day. If you smile and have your head up, it becomes another type of therapy: seeking happiness everywhere!

Pleasure: Giving and Receiving with Gratitude

One of the MVPs that really helped me was the practice of being intentional about gratitude. It's way too easy for me to get focused on the difficulty of my daily regimen, the slow progress that happens at times, or the fairly regular renegotiations of the medication protocol. But just 5 or 10 minutes focused on all of the beautiful people in my life and the progress I have made is so helpful to sustain a positive life, day in and day out.

In the Third Quarter chapter, we discussed happiness as one of my goals for 2014. One of the significant points was to find opportunities for "random acts of kindness." This is the ultimate giving trait, when you do not expect anything in return. It is purely kindness to another person, whether it is an adult, child, an elderly person, or a group, that did not expect or ask for something. Kindness does not expect anything in return.

The other characteristic of happiness is receiving, which can be anything from emotional support, love, forgiveness, or just helpfulness. The key to finding happiness in receiving is gratitude! We have received loads of support along the journey dealing with Parkinson's and now is the time to acknowledge what others have given with their advice, knowledge, and compassion. I make it a point to thank those who provide even little things, like giving me a Kleenex when I am having drops put in my eye and cannot find the tissue with my eyes closed. Just that simple word "Thanks!" builds and feeds us emotionally.

Looking back at how unselfish people have been on my behalf is moving, and their support can never be repaid.

The Bob Team provided the guidance to continue fighting Parkinson's, and it was with their help that I now have *The Parkinson's Playbook* that we've developed over the last five years. Each team member played a key part of "A Game Plan to Put Your Parkinson's on the Defense." I feel intense gratitude for each of their contributions to improving my quality of life.

To acknowledge the contributions of each would take an Overtime Quarter. I will leave it simply as "Thank You."

I'M WINNING THIS GAME!

By the end of the Fourth Quarter, you have a frame of reference on Parkinson's from a physical standpoint and what it takes to stay in the game. In the First Quarter, you pulled together your defense coach and team lineup to put together all of the best plays. In the Second Quarter, you started to work on your offense, incorporating fitness, supplements, nutrition, and alternative therapies that can dramatically improve your results. In the Third Quarter, you started to track that scoreboard and all of your progress. And now in this Fourth Quarter, you have decided who your MVPs are and given them the plays and strategies you need to support your mental and emotional well-being. Fitness, medications, supplements, and muscular therapy can be quantified, but the emotional and mental management of the disease will be a constantly evolving learning process.

The good news is that you have begun to take control of your life and develop the personal commitment to move the game forward on offense. All of your coaches, players, and MVPs are necessary, and it's incredibly important to not lean too heavily on one over the others. Balance is the key. The more you can do on your own, the more it will lead to happiness and enjoying life's treasures.

As time runs out on the Fourth Quarter, you are a completely different person has and have evolved for the better from the beginning

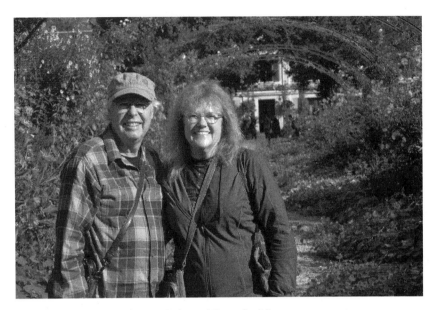

Bob and Jean Smith

of the game. This one singular victory is the time to celebrate your accomplishments and laurels, but do not become complacent. The season is ongoing, and you will continue to meet your match with the Parkinson's team; but now you have the tools to start developing the Game Plan for the upcoming game and all of the future games.

SWEET VICTORY!

What follows is the conversation that took place during the concluding session with my psychologist.

"Bob, you have come so far," he started. "Look at you. Physically, you barely present any Parkinson's symptoms; and emotionally, you're a far cry from the angry, bitter, and frightened man who walked into my office not too long ago."

"Thank you. Yes, I feel stronger, physically and emotionally. I still have some really tough days and weeks, but generally I'm feeling good, and life is getting a little better every day." I smiled, noticing the difference in my body all these years later. My heart was beating happily. I was breathing easier. My posture was better and more relaxed in the chair. *Yes ... there have definitely been some big wins.*

"I've really enjoyed helping you, and I hope you'll keep in touch."

"Actually, I'd like to plan on meeting up with you again regularly. It would be good for me to check in and make sure that I answer those questions—what am I doing for mastery? What am I doing for pleasure?—at least every few months. Having you on my team has helped so much. Your insight and support have really helped me shift my attitude, my behaviors, and my relationships for the better. I know this is the end of our current plan, but I'm going to be on the field with Parkinson's for a long time," I said matter-of-factly.

"I have really enjoyed being on your team. And yes, please count on me to jump onto the field with you to celebrate or problem-solve," he said as he reached out to shake my hand.

As I walked to the car this time, I felt such relief and gratitude wash over me.

I am so grateful to have him and all of the other coaches and players in my life.

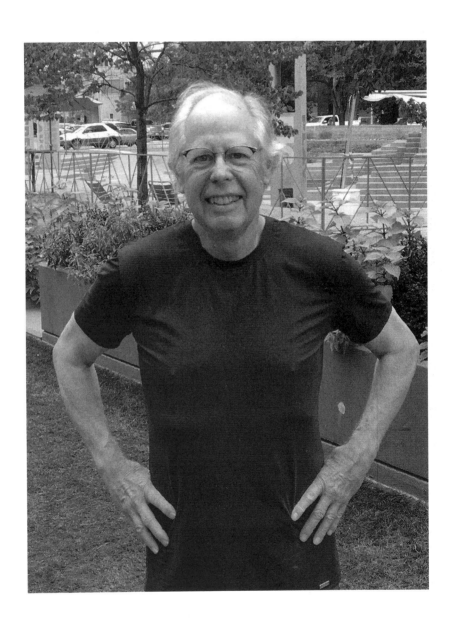

CONCLUSION:

VICTORY DANCE IN THE END ZONE

"Twenty, fifteen...no one can touch him...the crowd is screaming...will he make it to the End Zone before the clock runs out?" The announcer himself is almost screaming with excitement.

And then, "Touch-dooooooooooooown!"

The crowd gets on their feet, cheering and watching the player as he throws the ball down with excitement and begins his victory dance.

All of the players and coaches rush the field, butt-slapping, high-fiving, and hugging.

The game is won, and it's time to celebrate before they hit the field to train for the next one.

THE NEXT GAME

The opponent for the next game is always Team Parkinson's. It never changes, and the regularity is unrelenting. Every single day, you are reminded of that team's ability to attack your body and mind. When a time out is taken, it becomes a step backwards. *The Parkinson's Playbook* has outlined tools from traditional medicine and self-healing strategies to help you hold the line with Parkinson's.

Slowing down this disease takes a commitment to exercise and living healthfully in body and mind. The need for a training routine is essential in keeping you fit and flexible, creating the foundation for a fuller and more vibrant lifestyle. Keeping exercise as the most important part of your daily life is necessary to always stay a step ahead of this chronic disease. I am not sure how many seasons there will be in my career, but retirement is off in the distance with *The Parkinson's Playbook* by my side.

The Most Valuable Players on your team will always be there for support, so stay connected to them and follow their advice.

The next game is not about myself. It's about helping others. As I was writing this book, people would ask, "How is it coming? Are you done?" They see change and a healthy appearance, so there must be something to what I am doing. Friends and others with Parkinson's have been anxious for insight into this chronic disease and the plays they are missing that could help them turn the tide of their own game. They need something to believe in—something that will provide an avenue for change in their own life. *The Parkinson's Playbook* has changed my life, and I hope it will do the same for others.

The next game is about to kick off.

Stay committed!

APPENDIX:
YOGA POSES AND
EXERCISE ROUTINES

The following yoga routines were developed specifically for me by a yoga therapist relative to my fitness level.

Consult with a professional trainer before using any of the elements listed in these programs. The programs are strictly a guide for your yoga therapist as to what might be appropriate based on ability, and should be modified for physical limitations. Read about the different poses in one of the reference books in the Resources section (page 153) to get a better handle on the elements of the programs. Another option is to use a yoga video to get started.

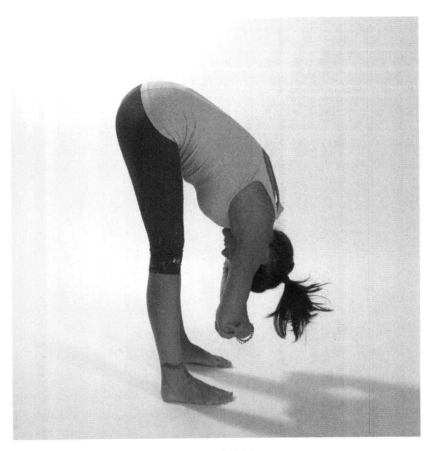

Forward Fold

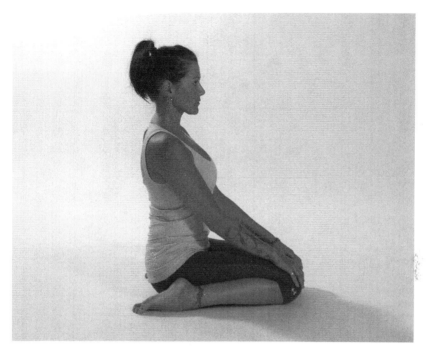

Meditation: Seated

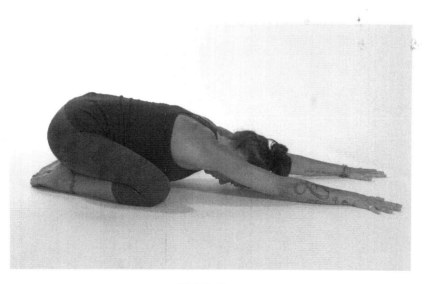

Child's Pose

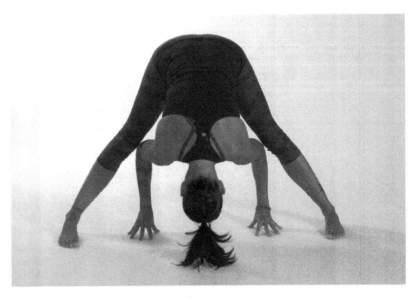

Wide-Legged Forward Fold

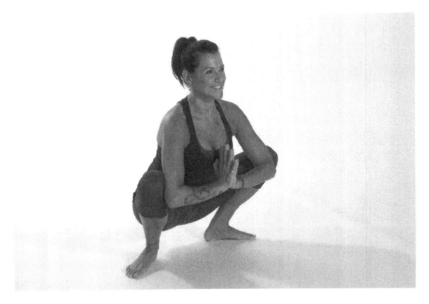

Horse Stance

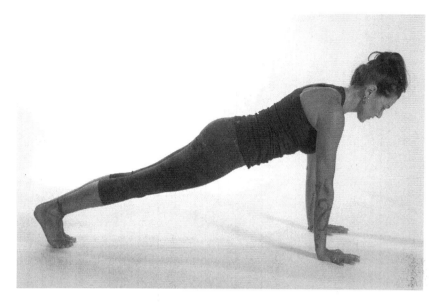

Plank

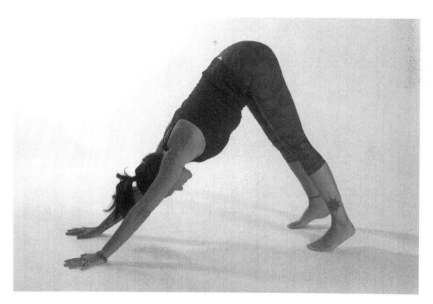

Downward Facing Dog

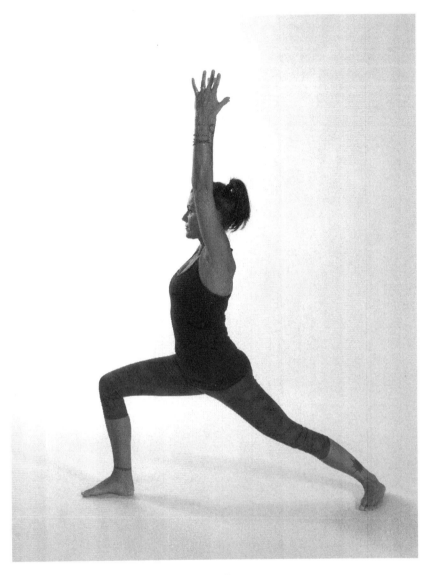

Crescent Lunge

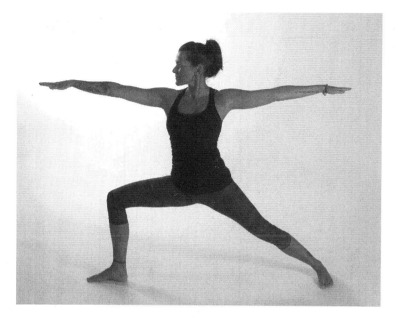

Warrior Two

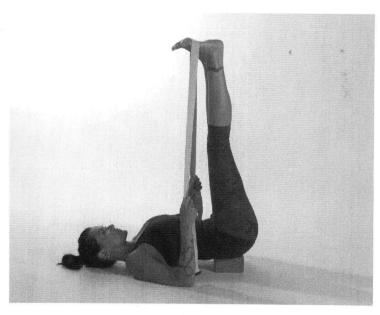

Leg Extension

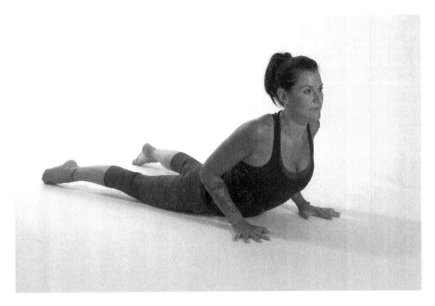

Preparing for Cobra Pose

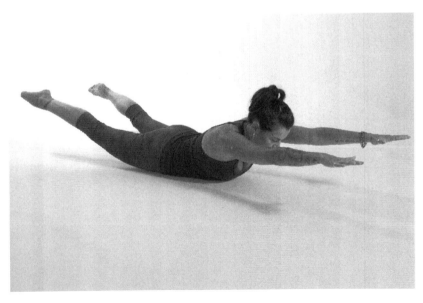

Locust

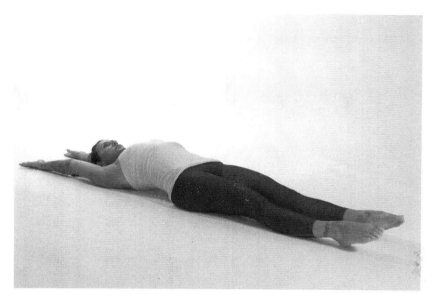

Preparation for Bridge Pose

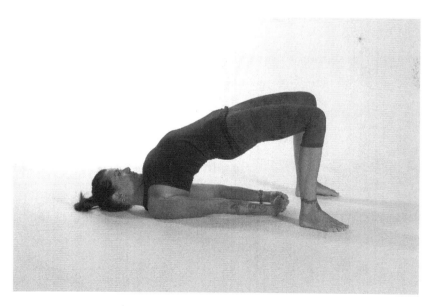

Bridge

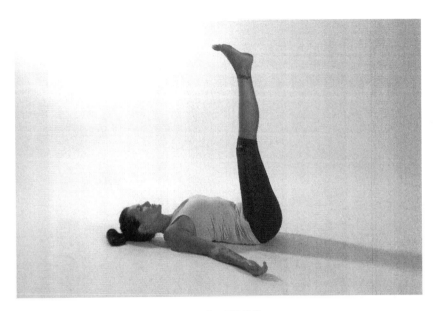

Feet-up-the-Wall Pose

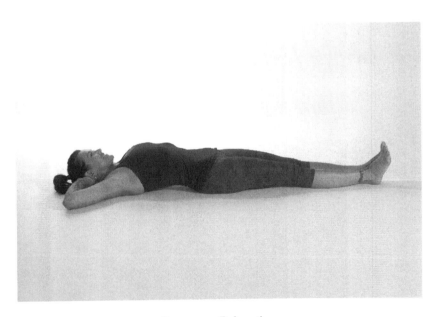

Savasana: Relaxation

EXERCISE ROUTINE 1: OVERALL FLEXIBILITY AND FITNESS

- Begin with stretching and flexibility, incorporating some of the following joint freeing exercises:

  - Mountain pose (hands overhead); back bend with arms like goal posts; forward fold.

  - Sitting on your heels using your backside or a block to reach a comfortable position, do a wrist and arm joint freeing series with the arms outstretched (flex and point the hands and make circles in both directions with hands clenched) while also stretching the thighs.

  - Sitting with the legs outstretched, do the foot and leg joint freeing series (flex and point the feet and make circles in both directions).

- Start with a cardio routine for twenty minutes, using any combination of elliptical machine, stationary bike, or treadmill.

- Balance work on the bosu ball with bare feet: Step-ups on the bosu ball alternating right and left, stepping up then down. Next step up on the opposite side of the ball, turn around, and repeat. Step up and balance with both feet on the ball and squat down, keep practicing at each session until you can squat down ten times.

- Tree pose.

- Crescent lunge with dumbbell: alternating opening the arms, repeating five times with each arm without losing balance.

- Repeat crescent lunge with the eyes open and turning the head side to side (only after you can do the regular crescent lunge five times in a row).

- Chest openers for spinal strengthening.

- Armless cobra (arms stay down).

- Locust pose (with the arms bound behind the back), lift the chest and legs.

- Bridge pose: squeeze a block between the knees, lift the hips, and press the feet and head down.

- Cooling down: Lying down on your back, bring the knees to the chest and squeeze using both arms (give yourself a big hug).

- Still lying down with knees down, twist to the left, return to center, then twist to the right; repeat three times.

- Savasana: Lying down, with your arms by your side, rest to clear your mind.

EXERCISE ROUTINE 2:
CORE STRENGTH, BALANCE, AND FLEXIBILITY

- Use the startup cardio and stretching routines previously described in Exercise Routine 1.

- Abdominal exercise routine. A combination of sit-ups and crunches, first with legs bent and arms behind your head, then with legs raised and bending at the waist.

- Bent knee crunches with ball between knees. Begin in a striding position with the ball between the knees. Lower the back knee towards the floor with the front knee bent. Raise up and step forward, then repeat by striding forward and beginning over.

- Forearm plank. First get in a push-up position, then lower your forearms to the floor and hold.

- Plank to Downward Dog sequence. Start with the push-up position then raise your bottom to a V-shape pose with your feet on the balls of your feet. Transition back to a plank.

- Crescent lunge pose. Start in a standing stride positon and bend the front leg to 90 degrees, keeping the back leg straight. Raise both hands over your head.

- Warrior pose. Start with the crescent lunge position, with one arm pointing forward and the other arm pointing back. Look forward at the front hand.

- Horse Stance. With the legs wide, fold forward and reach down and hold each ankle or foot.

- Seated twist pose. Begin by sitting on the mat with both legs extended. Bring one leg in to a 90 degree position and turn your body to the side, while the hand opposite to the bent leg grabs the knee and gently pulls the leg in. The opposite arm is palm-side down on the floor.

- Cool-down and Savasana. Lay flat on the mat with both legs extended, arms by your side, palms up, and eyes closed.

EXERCISE ROUTINE 3:
BALANCE AND FLEXIBILITY

- Tools: block, bead chanting ring ("Mala"), and strap.

- Mountain pose: with a block between the feet (big toes touching, not the heels, keeping the feet parallel).

- Standing forward bend: Bend with a block between the shins (big toes point in, heels wide or weight on the balls of the feet).

- Armless cobra (block between feet or the shins, with toes pressing down): lift the chest with the elbows bent. On the second set, lift the chest and legs.

- Seated twist: cross one lifted knee over the lower bent knee and twist the opposite shoulder toward the top of the knee.

- Meditation: Sit up tall and close the eyes, using a breath awareness technique such as chanting "so" on the inhale and "hum" on the exhale; the length of time should increase until a full rotation has been made with the chanting beads.

- Note: this program should be done five times a week and is in addition to any other exercise class.

RESOURCES

ONLINE RESOURCES

Parkinson's Association of the Rockies
  (www.parkinsonrockies.org)

National Parkinson's Foundation
  (www.parkinson.org)

Michael J. Fox Foundation
  (www.michaeljfox.org)

Davis Phinney Foundation
  (www.davisphinneyfoundation.org)

GetFitNow.com

SUGGESTED READINGS AND REFERENCES

Christina Brown, *Ten Minute Yoga for Flexibility and Focus*
Great book that highlights flexibility, which is so important for those with Parkinson's.

Suza Francina, *The New Yoga for Healthy Aging*
A yoga book that relates well to the exercise needs for those with physical limitations.

Shakta Kaur Khalsa, *Kundalini Yoga*
A useful guide for understanding yoga poses and their benefits in your fitness program.

Gwen Lawrence, *Body Sculpting with Yoga*
This book offers a combination of yoga movements with light strength-building workouts and endurance exercises.

Yoga Journal Magazine
I like this magazine because you can create your own yoga sequences and workouts.

FINDING A BOWEN AND SCENAR PRACTITIONER

Bowen therapists can now be found around the globe. Many medical practitioners are incorporating Bowen therapy as a viable alternative for self-healing treatment versus traditional medicine. When my Bowen therapist relocated, I searched the Internet for people with the skills and background to continue this treatment strategy. It took several phone conversations with potential Bowen practitioners to find one in my region capable of providing similar Bowen treatment who had the qualifications to fit my needs. I found a therapist an hour's drive from home. I would also suggest having a friend drive you to and from a session, as your body will be making adjustments after a treatment. Bowen Practitioners can be found through www.ibowen.ca (worldwide directory) and www.bowendirectory.com (predominantly a U.S. directory)

Finding a SCENAR practitioner is a little more problematic. Since it is a newer and lesser known treatment strategy, it can be harder to find a local qualified practitioner. I have found several companies on the Internet that manufacture SCENAR devices for home use. My suggestion is that you research them thoroughly before going down this path. My approach would be to search for groups that offer natural healing alternatives. Another source of practitioners might be to contact the companies that manufacture SCENAR devices and ask for recommendations for those who might practice in your area.

ABOUT THE AUTHOR

Robert W. Smith's professional roots evolved from a forty-year career as a landscape architect in Denver, Colorado. He was recognized as a leader, mentor, teacher, community activist, and environmental steward, and inducted as a Fellow in the American Society of Landscape Architects for a legacy of innovative design and community service.

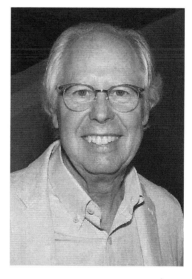

Drawing upon his dormant passion for helping others in need and combining it with a playbook that has literally changed his life, Robert has embarked on a second career as an author and speaker. His mission is to provide a ray of hope for those suffering with Parkinson's, a debilitating disease of unknown origin and cure.